Shakhlo Bakieva
Tulkin Bobojonov

IMPACT OF BLOOD DISEASES ON THE COURSE OF

Shakhlo Bakieva
Tulkin Bobojonov

IMPACT OF BLOOD DISEASES ON THE COURSE OF

AND TREATMENT OF RHINOSINUSITIS

ScienciaScripts

Cover image: www.ingimage.com

This book is a translation from the original published under ISBN 978-3-659-90607-7.

Publisher:
Sciencia Scripts
is a trademark of
Dodo Books Indian Ocean Ltd. and OmniScriptum S.R.L publishing group

120 High Road, East Finchley, London, N2 9ED, United Kingdom
Str. Armeneasca 28/1, office 1, Chisinau MD-2012, Republic of Moldova, Europe
Managing Directors: Ieva Konstantinova, Victoria Ursu
info@omniscriptum.com

Printed at: see last page
ISBN: 978-620-8-37055-8

Contents

The monograph covers etiopathogenetic, genetic, clinical and diagnostic aspects of adenoiditis in frequently ill children and approaches to complex treatment.
The monograph is intended for otolaryngologists, doctoral students, masters and clinical residents.

Abdullaeva N.N. - Doctor of medical sciences, associate professor of "Otorhinolaryngology" department, Tashkent Medical Academy;
Vokhidov U.N. - Doctor of Medical Sciences, Associate Professor

CHAPTER 1

Modern ideas about etiology, pathogenesis and treatment of inflammatory diseases of the nose and paranasal sinuses

In recent years there has been a significant increase in the number of diseases of the nose and paranasal sinuses (NNPS). According to S.Z. Piskunov and G.Z. Piskunov (2005), the number of sinusitis cases per 1000 people increased from 4.6 to 12.2 between 2000 and 2004 [54]. During this time interval, the number of patients with MNiONP increased annually by 1.5-2% and reached 52.7%. From 2005 to 2015, patients hospitalised for paranasal sinus diseases accounted for approximately 2/3 of the total number of patients in specialised hospitals. In Uzbekistan, the incidence of MNiONP is 65-70% and tends to increase [52]. This is associated with significant air pollution with various ecotoxicants, a significant decrease in the immune system of the macroorganism, a high frequency of mixt-infections leading to the development of purulent inflammatory process in the paranasal sinuses and the development of antibiotic resistance.

In addition, there is a tendency to a prolonged course of sinusitis, rapid spread of infection to the lower respiratory tract. These diseases often cause the development of aphonic bronchitis, pneumonia or bronchial asthma, since the upper and lower respiratory tracts constitute morphologically and functionally a unified system, and only in this way should it be considered in the treatment of diseases. The number of rhinosinuso- genic orbital and intracranial complications, often leading to disability or death of the patient, is not decreasing.The trigger in the development of rhinosinusitis is usually a viral infection.

An increase in morbidity is usually observed in autumn and spring, as well as during influenza epidemics. It is estimated that 10 million people in Russia suffer from acute rhinosinusitis annually. According to R.E.Gliklichand R.Metson (2005), rhinosinusitis considerably reduces the quality of life of people

[85] Studies in recent decades have shown that approximately 10% of rhinosinusitis is odontogenic in nature. One of the possible pathogenetic factors in the development of recurrent rhinosinusitis in children is gastroesophageal reflux and pharyngolaryngeal reflux, which causes significant inhibition of mucociliary transport (MTT) of the nasal mucosa.

According to the classification of V.S. Kozlov (2003) and LundV.etal. (2000) [98]rhinosinusitis is divided into the following forms:

- ***Acute*** (sinus inflammation lasting no more than 8 weeks)

in adults and not more than 12 weeks in children);

- ***recurrent acute*** (2-4 episodes of acute sinusitis within a year separated by asymptomatic intervals);
- ***subacute*** (characterised by the manifestation of mild to severe sinusitis symptoms without acute respiratory infection and without abrupt worsening during

the course of the disease);

- ***chronic*** (persistence of inflammation in the sinuses for more than 8-12 weeks, in addition, this diagnosis is revealed if there is no improvement after 4 weeks from the start of drug therapy, and changes in the mucous membrane in the sinuses are confirmed by computed tomography);
- ***exacerbation of chronic*** (worsening of usual symptoms and/or

the appearance of new symptoms).

The microflora of the nasal cavity of healthy people is represented mainly by micrococci, staphylococci, Neisseria.In sinusitis, there is an increase in microbial contamination of the nasal mucosa, and not only pathogenic but also opportunistic microbes are isolated. The main bacterial causative agents of rhinosinusitis (in 70% of cases) are Str. pneumoniae and Haemofhilusinfluenzae.Y some patients sowing from the nasal cavity and sinuses is sterile, which is explained by the presence of viral or anaerobic flora, resistant to traditionally used antibiotics, the possibility of the presence of which is often not taken into account. At exacerbation of the chronic process, the spectrum of pathogens changes significantly, but among the pathogens are also present Str. pneumoniae (2-7%), H. influenzae (9-24%), Str. pyogenes (9-10%) and Staph, aureus (6-16%). Dental diseases (odontogenic maxillary sinusitis) may also play a role in the aetiology of maxillary sinusitis. In recent years, the role of chlamydia in the etiology of rhinosinusitis has been discussed.

An effective physiological barrier and filter preventing the entry of infectious agents into the body is the mucous membrane of the upper respiratory tract with the presence of mucociliary clearance and immune defence. Thanks to mucociliary clearance occurs self-cleansing of the respiratory tract. It has a leading role in maintaining homeostasis of the upper respiratory tract and the respiratory system as a whole. Mucus transport in the nasal cavity depends on two factors - the activity of the crescentic mucous membranes of the mucociliary epithelium and the production of nasal secretion. The mucociliary transport system (MTS) consists of three components:

- The superficial mesenteric and secreting epithelium;
- glands of the intrinsic layer of the mucous membrane;
- mucus produced by these glands and bocaloid cells.

The ratio of mesenteric and bocaloid cells is 1:5. The decisive factor for the introduction of microorganisms into the mucous membrane of the nasal cavity is the death or dysfunction of the mesenteric epithelium; genetic defects (primary cilia dyskinesia, Carta-Guéner syndrome, Young's syndrome), exposure to viruses or bacterial toxins may themselves become an important pathogenetic factor. In acute purulent sinusitis in children, there is a significant prolongation of the saccharine test time to 10.84±0.49 min and a decrease in the motor activity of the ciliary apparatus of the nasal mucosa to 0.34±0.26 Hz in the lower nasal cavity and 3.42±2.17 Hz in the middle nasal cavity.

An important protective factor is mucus secreted by bocaloid cells and epitheliocytes, which comes to the surface of the mucous membrane constantly, as their secretory activity is carried out asynchronously under the influence of local irritating factors. The composition of mucus includes: mucin, secreted by mucous cells, as well as possessing antibacterial activity lysozyme, lactoferrin and secretory IgA. Non-specific factors include: mucus glycoproteins (fu- comycins, sialomycins, sulphomycins), which have pronounced bacteriostatic and bactericidal abilities; lysozymes secreted by serous cells; lactoferrin, secreted by serous cells, which transports iron ions into the bacterial cell and thus has antioxidant activity; secretory glucosidases, interferon, complement (enzyme system), secretory proteases; phagocytic system, which includes mononuclear phagocytes and polymorphonuclear leukocytes. Specific factors are represented by recognition (receptors of T and B-lymphocytes) or effector (antibodies) molecules, have a common origin, contain similar amino acid sequences, belong to the immunoglobulin family and play a role of defence against invading microorganisms.

Significantly more IgG than IgA is detected in paranasal sinus secretions. Perhaps circulating antibodies are of greater importance to the paranasal sinus mucosa due to the highly efficient local blood flow. It is assumed that relative insufficiency of secretory antibodies in the sinus region determines the tendency to recurrent course of sinusitis due to inhibition of mucociliary clearance.

The most important form of communication between the organism and the external environment, which does not cease throughout the human life, is communication through the respiratory system. Nasal breathing is a normal physiological act and its disruption can cause functional and morphological shifts in the vital activity and structure of the most important organs and systems of the organism, which occur as a result of slowing down of metabolic processes, reduction of the bioelectric potential of the cell, the emergence of energy deficit due to oxygen deficiency, impaired microcirculation, as well as weakening of ciliary and epithelial functions. Switching off of nasal breathing leads to difficulties in venous outflow, which causes increased intracranial pressure and changes in cerebral vessels.

Anomalies of the intranasal structures and the lattice labyrinth are one of the main factors that impair the patency of the natural orifices of the paranasal sinuses and the mechanisms of their aeration and cleansing. These include anomalies in the development of the nasal shells, deviation of the nasal septum and deformation of the nasal valve. The pathological effect creates conditions for blockade of the ostiomeatal complex, and subsequently the development of inflammatory process in the paranasal sinuses. In conditions of stagnation of secretion and reduction of partial pressure of oxygen in the ENP, favourable conditions for the development of bacterial infection are created.

According to V.V. Shilenkova (2010), as the child grows, there is a change in the main indicators of nasal breathing in the form of an increase in total volume flow and a decrease in nasal resistance, with no significant sex differences [71]. In inflammatory processes in the paranasal sinuses, the periodicity of fluctuations is shorter than in the norm, but their species identity is preserved, which allows us to consider the nasal cycle as a persistent physiological phenomenon reflecting the reactivity of the nasal cavity mucosa.

Full-fledged realisation of nasal functions is a necessary condition not only for the absence of diseases of ENT organs (paranasal sinuses, middle ear, pharynx), but also for a sufficient quality of life of a modern person.

The study of nasal function is a mandatory condition for the preparation of rhinological patients for surgical or conservative treatment. One of the main criteria of treatment effectiveness is the determination of nasal respiratory function.

Of all the variety of techniques, the more objective and reliable can be considered those that provide for simultaneous determination of two indicators - pressure in the nasal cavity and the volume velocity of air flow arising from it, that is, they allow to obtain the value of nasal resistance, reflecting the degree of narrowing of the nasal passages [illegible]. Modern devices allow to determine the volume of air flow, as well as the difference in pressure between the nasal vestibule and the nasopharynx. It is now possible to quantify the parameters, store them in the computer memory, and compare the parameters during the entire period of patient observation. The results of computerised pneumotachymetry in patients with sinusitis showed a direct correlation between subjective sensations and objective indicators of nasal breathing. Acoustic rhinometry is a fundamentally new approach to assessing the state of the nasal cavity, which allows to determine the cross-sectional area and volumetric indices. However, acoustic rhinometry does not measure the flow of air jet and nasal breathing, it provides an opportunity to quantitatively characterise pathological changes in the nasal cavity.

Assessment of the state of the upper respiratory tract should include the study of the functional state of the nasal mucosa. The use of certain methods of research allows not only to assess the functional reserve of this most important biological barrier of the organism, but also to identify reliably enough this or that pathology, to carry out its directed treatment, to solve correctly the issues of prevention. They allow earlier diagnosis of MNIONP, as functional disorders in the upper respiratory tract develop much earlier than morphological ones. Currently, many researchers recommend saccharin test as the simplest and most informative method of ICTS research.

Significant scientific and practical results in the study of the transport function of the nasal mucosal epithelium were obtained by Piskunov S.Z. et al. [53]; Pluzhnikov M.S. (2002) [57]; PuchellG., (2005) [102]; ProcktorD.F. (2007) [101]. Thus, PassaliD. etal., (2000) [100] determined the time of mucous layer replacement over the epithelial surface: on the posterior 2/3 surfaces of the mucosa this time is 10 minutes, and on the anterior 1/3 - within one hour [101]. H. Riechelmannetal., (2008) also investigated the frequency of cilia beating [107].

Thus, in diseases of the nose and paranasal sinuses the transport function of the mesenteric epithelium is disturbed. The study of this function in the dynamics is a highly informative criterion for determining the quality of treatment, both surgical and conservative S.Z. Piskunov (2010). The suction function of the nose was investigated by applying turundas moistened with 1% atropine solution to the nasal mucosa. According to Makronosov M.A., Tarasov G.D. (2012), when both respiratory and transport functions are disturbed, the suction function accelerated in a directly proportional relationship [47].

One of the most important functions performed by the nasal mucosa is the protective function. Its manifestation is accompanied by changes in local and general reactivity, one of the indicators of which is temperature. Violation of nasal breathing contributes to an increase in the contact time of these factors with the mucous membrane, causing inflammation, which is accompanied by a temperature response.Olfactory analyser is an important information channel that provides communication with the surrounding world.

Olfaction depends not only on the state of the olfactory cleft and the entire olfactory area, but also on the state of the nasal cavity mucosa, the degree of its blood filling, temperature, and excretory capacity. However, the existing methods of objective assessment of nasal functions do not allow for a detailed characterisation of the subjective sensations of rhino- logical patients, the degree of influence of the disease on their general well-being, performance and social role.

Diagnosis of sinusitis often does not cause special problems: the presence of facial pain, difficulty in nasal breathing, purulent discharge from the nose and smell disorders make the patient turn to a doctor and carry out the necessary examination and treatment in a timely manner. Pain is more often localised in the frontal region, less often - in the projection zone of the maxillary sinus. However, in children, the symptoms and manifestations of sinusitis are rarely specific. The main complaints, as a rule, are prolonged runny nose, persistent cough that increases on waking, nasality, difficulty in nasal breathing, general weakness, prolonged subfebrile, loss of appetite and rapid fatigue.

Headache is observed rarely and mainly in children over 10 years of age. The incidence of pain syndrome in acute sinusitis in paediatric practice ranges from 29% to 33%, while rhinorrhoea is observed in 71-80% of cases and cough in 83% of children.

The peculiarities of the clinical course of acute sinusitis in childhood create certain problems in the differential diagnosis of this disease with allergic rhinitis, which is also accompanied by swelling of the mucous membrane of the ONP, sometimes even significant. Therefore, despite the presence of typical complaints indicating a possible lesion of the ONP, the doctor is faced with a dilemma. Is it an uncomplicated upper respiratory tract infection, allergic rhinitis or sinus infection?

There is no doubt that otorhinolaryngologists, especially outpatient specialists, as well as family doctors and paediatricians, should have an accurate diagnostic method that can identify ONP lesions and distinguish them from respiratory infections, chronic adenoiditis, allergic and vasomotor rhinitis. In addition, the method should be able to be used repeatedly in the process of dynamic monitoring of the patient without compromising health.

The most common and widespread method of investigation in acute sinusitis is *review radiography of the* ONP. For topical diagnosis of paranasal sinus lesions, direct projections (nasolabial, nasolabial and frontal) and lateral axial projection are most often used. V.S. Kozlov in his monograph "Inflammation of the nasal sinuses in children" (2006, 2007) wrote: "Summarising the data obtained during radiological examination in different projections, it is possible to obtain valuable information about the anatomo-topographical relations of the sinuses, their shape and size" [40]. [40].

However, radiography in several projections represents a large radiation load for the child, which is undoubtedly one of the significant disadvantages of the method. In addition, as a result of the relief of the facial skeleton, interpretation of the information obtained during radiography is very difficult.

Many authors question the reliability and specificity of review radiography. R.P.Luck (2006) performed a radiological study of the ONP with sinusitis symptoms and compared the findings with computed tomography (CT) [97]. The concordance of both studies was observed in only 74% of cases. According to studies by other authors, the specificity of plain radiography is lower, ranging from 23% to 63%.

Failures in the use of native radiography are also explained by the fact that decreased pneumatisation of the ONP on the radiograph does not give the opportunity to judge with complete reliability about the nature of the pathological process in the sinuses. Only the presence of a clear horizontal level indicates the presence of pathological secretion in the sinus. It should be noted the low specificity of review radiography in the diagnosis of ethmoiditis, frontitis and sphenoiditis. In this regard, many authors consider review radiography as an insufficiently reliable method of recognising sinusitis. According to the "European position on rhinosinusitis and nasal polyps" published in the international journal "Rhinology" in 2005 and 2007, native radiography is not considered a mandatory examination and is excluded from the diagnostic algorithm in diseases of the ENP, especially in children.

In the last two decades, *computed tomography (CT)* has become a recognised method of diagnosing paranasal sinusitis. It is considered appropriate to perform the study in coronal projection, which provides maximum information about the state of the ostiomeatal complex, and axial projection, which provides visualisation of the cuneiform sinus and the location of such important anatomical structures as the oculomotor nerves, internal carotid artery, and orbit. CT provides a spatial representation of the relationship between intranasal structures and the ONP, allows to judge the nature of anatomical disorders and their influence on the development of the pathological process, to assess the characteristic of tissues by their X-ray density and differentiate mucosal oedema from polyps and cysts, serve as a map for planning surgical intervention and a guide for the surgeon during surgery.Despite the obvious advantages, CT has some disadvantages. According to the "European Position on Rhinosinusitis and Nasal Polyps. CT of the ONP should not be considered as the first step in the diagnostic algorithm for acute and recurrent sinusitis, nor for exacerbation of chronic non-polyposis. A thorough history and nasal endoscopy are considered sufficient in these cases.

Currently, *optical endoscopy* is considered to be one of the leading methods of diagnostics of ENT pathology. Visibility of the endoscopic method, its high informativeness allow obtaining reliable information about the state of those parts of the nasal cavity, which are inaccessible during conventional examination and traditional methods of examination. Taking into account the effectiveness and low invasiveness of endoscopy, most authors consider it to be the most promising technique and recommend to include it in the standard diagnostic algorithm. However, most of the studies devoted to the optical method of diagnosis address the issues of endoscopy application for the detection of chronic pathology of the nasal cavity and nasopharynx.

It is emphasised that endoscopic examination is intended to detect various variants of the anatomical structure of the lateral wall of the nasal cavity and nasal septum, predisposing to the development of a long-term inflammatory process in the ENP. Detection of pathological discharge in the ostiomeatal complex is a reliable criterion for the diagnosis of sinusitis. However, not always signs of sinusitis can be detected endoscopically. Having performed endoscopy of the middle and upper nasal passages in 100 patients with sinusitis, S.S. Limansky and O.V. Kondrasheva (2005) were able to diagnose sinusitis only in 81 cases [44].

Ultrasound (USG) is based on the principle of ultrasound waves travelling through the tissues of the body and reflecting at the boundary of media that differ in density. In fact, there are two different ways of recording ultrasound reflections at the boundary of different tissues when examining the ONP:

1) A-scan, or one-dimensional ultrasound. In foreign literature this method is known as "A-mode", in domestic literature as A-method and

2) B-scan, or two-dimensional ultrasound. Synonyms: B-mode, B-mode, B-method, echotomography, two-dimensional ultrasonography, sinus sonography, sonography.The results of ultrasound of the ONP have been compared with the gold standard such as lavage of the maxillary sinus for puncture and of the frontal sinus for anterior fracture. Ultrasound is a reliable method of detecting exudative sinusitis. The concordance of ultrasound and review radiography, according to various authors, ranges from 80 to 95%, 74% for radiography and anthroscopy, and 75% for anthroscopy and ultrasound. T.Puhakka et al (2000) conducted a comparative analysis of sensitivity and specificity of review radiography, NMR tomography and A- method of ultrasound in acute maxillary sinusitis in adults [103]. According to the author's data, the sensitivity of ultrasound was 86%, the specificity of the method was 95%. The concordance of ultrasound and radiography was observed in 80% of cases, ultrasound and NMR - in 64%. The author noted that the use of ultrasound significantly reduces the need to use radiological method in the diagnosis of inflammatory processes in the ENP. Cost-effectiveness, safety, high informativeness and simplicity determine the significant advantages of ultrasound as a screening method of diagnosis in the examination of patients with ENP pathology. V.V.Byrikhina (2007), having conducted a comparative analysis of one-dimensional, two-dimensional ultrasound and review radiography in adults, pointed out that the sensitivity of the A-method of ultrasound in chronic sinusitis with cysts and polyps is rather low and does not exceed 53.1%, accuracy - 54%, specificity - 35% [20]. In addition, the author emphasised the impossibility of studying the ethmoidal cells and wedge-shaped sinus with one-dimensional echolocation devices.As for two-dimensional ultrasound, there are only some reports in the literature about the use of this technique in sinusitis. However, the peculiarities of the anatomical structure of the ONP significantly limit the wide use of the method in the diagnosis of sinusitis; therefore, its detailed study is required.

A new breakthrough in optimising two-dimensional ultrasonography was made by German researchers H.Riechelmann and W.Mann 2008 [108].According to the authors, two-dimensional imaging of three-dimensional structures, such as the ONP, provides better topographic orientation and interpretation than the A-method of ultrasonography. Two-dimensional scanning has been shown to provide the ability to examine the orbit and laminapapyracea, especially when orbital structures are involved in inflammation, trauma or tumour process. In this regard, H. Riechelmann and W.Mann formulated the following indications for B-scanning of the ONP: inflammatory processes in the sinuses (sinusitis); traumatic changes (haematomas of soft tissues of the face, fractures of the anterior and lateral walls of the maxillary and frontal sinuses, prolapse of the orbital wall, haematoma of the sinus, orbit, fractures of the nasal bones and frontal processes of the maxilla); tumours, mucocele and foreign bodies of the paranasal sinuses; inflammatory processes, edema and tumours of soft tissues of the face, V.V.Byrikhina in 2007 conducted a comparative analysis of the informativity of overview radiography, one-dimensional and two-dimensional ultrasonography and CT in various pathologies of the ONP [20]. The author noted the high sensitivity and specificity of two-dimensional ultrasonography in chronic sinusitis and the informativeness of the method in detecting such pathological conditions as foreign bodies of the maxillary sinuses, osteomas, tumours and mucocele.

The introduction of endoscopic surgical techniques in otorhinolaryngology has created prerequisites for the search for new methods of surgical treatment. Microsurgical and endoscopic techniques (operating microscopes, endoscopes, high-speed drills and microdebriders) make it possible to make surgery minimally traumatic and as safe as possible, preserving the mucous membrane of natural openings. The most sparing in terms of physiology of the nasal mucosa are submucosal interventions. In recent years, new, less traumatic methods of surgery have appeared using laser treatment, cryoconchotomy, radio wave intervention, electron knife. The modern concept of functional endonasal surgery is based on new data on the physiology and pathophysiology of the mucous membrane of the nasal cavity and ONP, performing sparing, minimally invasive, organ-preserving interventions within the ostiomeatal complex. The gentle principle is realised in two directions on the line of anaesthesia and on the line of improvement of the operative technique itself. The applied tactics, the sequence of examination stages and the volume of surgical intervention are aimed, first of all, at preserving what has been created by nature during the long period of evolution of the human organism. This requires patient and caring care of the mucous membrane, endowed by nature with numerous functions aimed at protecting the organism, as well as giving surgical treatment a more preventive direction.

Therapy of recurrent inflammation of the nose and paranasal sinuses is not always effective. In addition, some antibiotics have the opposite of the desired immunosuppressive effect. In recent years, there is increasing evidence that most of the commonly used antibiotics have immunosuppressive effects. Since the violation of immune mechanisms is an obligatory link in the pathogenesis of various forms of purulent sinusitis, in modern conditions successful treatment is impossible without taking into account the mechanisms of the effect of drugs on the immune system of the patient. Moreover, the state of immunological resistance of the organism largely determines the course of this disease. In recent years, new methods of immune system correction have been developed. Currently used drugs can not only affect directly on the infectious agent, but also modulate the inflammatory process, induce local and general immune reactions. Immunotherapy has become especially important due to the increase of antibiotic-resistant strains among the causative agents of ENT-infections and the increasing role of opportunistic microbial flora in the etiology of ENT diseases.Modern immunomodulators are conditionally divided into three groups depending on their origin (microbial, chemical and biological): bacterial lysates (bronchomunal, IRS-19); membrane fractions (Biostim); bacterial ribosomes stimulated by membrane fractions (ribomunil).

The main directions of treatment of acute and recurrent sinusitis are eradication of the pathogen, as well as restoration of normal aeration of the ENP and mucociliary clearance of the mucosa. However, there is still no consensus on antibiotic therapy, as in 33% of children with acute sinusitis the infectious agent is not detected, and in 70% of cases positive dynamics is observed without the use of antibiotics. Children with recurrent sinusitis, as a rule, belong to the group of frequently ill children. Prolonged and repeated use of antibiotics can lead to the development of dysbacteriosis, allergies and other side effects. Therefore, there are more and more frequent reports in the literature about the need to limit the use of systemic antibiotic therapy.

An alternative treatment is local treatment of the ONP. However, there are controversial issues in this problem as well. Such techniques include the NMIC method based on the creation of controlled negative pressure in the nasal cavity. In the studies of V.V. Shilenkova (2008) showed that the negative pressure created in the nasal cavity during NMIC-procedure does not significantly affect the functional state of the nasal cavity [71]. After application of sinuscatheter there is no persistent inhibition of mucociliary transport and motor activity of the mesenteric epithelium, which can serve as a proof of safety of the NMIC method. NMIC method has not only high efficiency (96.9%) in the treatment of acute and recurrent sinusitis, but also significantly reduces the time of sanation of the paranasal sinuses. In mild to moderate sinusitis, including cases of ineffectiveness of systemic antibiotic therapy, the NMIC method is indicated as monotherapy. In severe, uncomplicated forms of the disease, the use of NMIC sinuscatheter in combination with systemic antibiotic therapy is optimal.

Summarising the above, it should be emphasised that puncture method of sinusitis treatment, drainage and probing of the ONP are rather complicated manipulations requiring high qualification of the doctor and in some cases anaesthesia in view of the peculiarities of psycho-emotional status. The invasiveness of these interventions does not exclude the occurrence of complications in oncohematological patients. Fear of puncture make them refuse the manipulation, which does not allow timely adequate treatment. Due to the above disadvantages, they can not be used in patients with severe haematological diseases and in children. This dictates the need to improve conservative methods of treatment in this category of patients.

1.2 Current understanding of the aetiology, pathogenesis and treatment of nasal haemorrhage

The problem of nasal haemorrhage (NB) does not lose its relevance. NB is the most common indication for emergency hospitalisation in ENT hospitals. The number of patients with NC admitted to specialised departments does not tend to decrease. The share of nosebleeds varies from 3 to 8% in the total structure of hospitalised patients. According to the materials of the ENT clinic of the Russian State Medical University on the basis of the multidisciplinary 1st City Clinical Hospital named after N.I. Pirogov. N.I. Pirogov Multidisciplinary 1st City Clinical Hospital named after N.I. Pirogov, patients with NK account for 14.3% of the total number of hospitalised patients and 20.5% of the emergency group [50].

Depending on the sources, localisation, time of onset, duration, causes of bleeding, various classifications of NK have been proposed. Most authors traditionally subdivide the causes of epistaxis into local, general and combined. In addition, bleeding is divided depending on the mechanism of occurrence into spontaneous and traumatic. From the type of damaged vessel: arterial, venous and capillary (microcirculatory). From the time of development: primary; early secondary, late secondary. Frequency of occurrence: sporadic and recurrent (recurrent). From clinical manifestations: manifest (external) and latent (internal or latent, such as haematosinus or haematoma). From the localisation of the source of bleeding: anteroposterior, posterior, superior, unilateral, bilateral. The volume of blood loss: minor (small, drop by drop), moderate, massive, profuse.

Predisposing factors also contribute to the development of NC: thinning and dryness of the nasal septum mucosa with subsequent ulceration in persons in contact with some chemical and other harmful substances;- presence of spikes and ridges on the deviated nasal septum, on which dystrophic changes in the mucosa develop;- ulceration and necrosis of nasal tissues due to specific inflammations, neoplasms (tuberculosis, lupus erythematosus, syphilis, cancer, sarcoma, etc.); - decreased resistance and pathology of the vascular wall; sudden changes in atmospheric pressure (in pilots, lupus erythematosus, syphilis, cancer, sarcoma, etc.).The combination of two or more predisposing factors favouring vascular rupture and bleeding significantly increases the risk of NK development.

Taking into account the etiological and pathogenetic diversity of NK, as well as the peculiarities of modern ideas about the mechanisms of hemorrhage development, the following clinical and pathogenetic classification is proposed:

I. Bleeding due to local destructive-necrotic processes of ENT organs.

1. New growths (malignant: cancer, sarcoma, etc.; benign: haemangiomas, angiofibromas of the nasal septum, juvenile angiofibroma of the nasopharynx, papillomas, etc.).

2. Granulomas and ulcers: in infectious lesions (tuberculosis, syphilis); in collagenoses (Wegener's granulomatosis, etc.).
3. Toxic and dystrophic lesions of ENT organs (chemical, thermal; in chronic diseases of ENT organs).
II. Bleeding of traumatic origin:
1. Vascular injuries in traumas and wounds (cut, chopped, gunshot, etc.).
2. Large vessel injuries during surgical interventions.
III. Bleeding due to an abnormality or lesion of the blood vessels:
1. Congenital vasopathies and mesenchymal dysplasias (hereditary telangiectasia (Randu-Osler disease); Marfan syndrome; local angiomatosis; Kazabach-Merritt syndrome (solitary hemangiomas with thrombocytopenia); carotid-cavernous junction and aneurysms of the internal carotid and other arteries).
2. Acquired vascular lesions (atherosclerosis; arterial hypertension: hypertension, symptomatic hypertension; vasculitis; angiopathies).
IV. Bleeding due to defects in the vascular and platelet link of haemostasis:
1. Thrombocytopenias (autoimmune; secondary).
2. Thrombocytopathies (hereditary thrombocytopathies; acquired (symptomatic) thrombocytopathies: drug-induced; renal failure; haemoblastosis, etc.).
3. Different types of Willebrand's disease.
V. Bleeding due to defects in coagulation haemostasis and fibrinolysis:
1. Hereditary coagulopathies: haemophilia A, B and C; hypopro-con- vertinemia; parahaemophilia; Stuart-Prower disease; hypoprothrombinemia; afibrinogenemia; dysfibrinogenemia; factor XIII deficiency.
2. Acquired coagulopathies: coagulopathies due to liver pathology; presence of immune inhibitors of factors Vili, IX, etc.; deficiency of K-vitamin-dependent factors II, VII, IX and X (during treatment with indirect anticoagulants, mechanical jaundice and intestinal dysbacteriosis); during consumption of clotting factors and platelets (DIC syndrome); during treatment with heparin.
3. Abnormalities of fibrinolysis due to the use of fibrinolytic drugs.

The presented clinical and pathogenetic classification of NK generalises the numerous clinical forms of this multifaceted and complex pathology, taking into account the variants of hemostasis system disorders and what disease this disorder is associated with.

Of course, this systematisation of causes, as well as other existing classifications, has a certain degree of conventionality, but it is convenient because it provides for differentiation of nosebleeds by pathogenesis and at the same time takes into account nosology. It can help the otorhinolaryngologist to understand the essence of complex disorders of the haemostasis system, facilitate their interpretation and subsequent correction, as well as reflect this pathology in a specific formulation of the diagnosis. This is very important because, firstly, special treatment is required for haemostasis abnormalities, and secondly, this or that dysfunction of the haemostasis system dictates the need for a number of measures, such as determining the duration of temporary disability, employment and so on.

Stopping bleeding from a damaged vessel requires the combined activity of platelet, vascular and humoral factors of blood plasma, balanced by the action of mechanisms that limit the accumulation of platelets and fibrin at the site of injury. Under physiological conditions, regulatory mechanisms prevent the uncontrolled development of blood coagulation. These mechanisms include removal of activated clotting factors from the blood by the liver, neutralisation of enzymes and activated cofactors in the blood. Of greatest importance is **antithrombin III, the** main inhibitor of key enzymes - thrombin, factors Xa and XIa. **The fibrinolytic** system is activated by the formation of fibrin. By dissolving fibrin, this system allows the lumen of the injured vessel to remain open; the equilibrium between fibrin formation and lysis ensures the preservation and renewal of the clot for several days, necessary for the healing of the injured vessel.

Treatment of ICH includes the solution of several problems: stopping bleeding, pathogenetically justified haemostatic and rational replacement therapy.Currently, there are many ways to stop ICH. However, in the practice of emergency care the most common method remains gauze tamponade of the nasal cavity. This method is simple, available for use at any stage of care and, in most cases, gives a quick effect. Gauze tampon allows you to tightly press the bleeding vessel. The mesh structure of the gauze acts as a "white clot" and accelerates the formation of a blood clot.

The disadvantages of gauze tamponade should, first of all, include activation of local fibrinolysis, which is a prerequisite for recurrences of NK. Insertion and removal of tampons is painful and can cause additional trauma to the nasal cavity mucosa, which leads to the formation of granulation tissue, which can also become a source of bleeding after tampon removal. Adhering to the mucous membrane, gauze tampons are quickly soaked with wound discharge and mucus, which creates conditions for the growth of microorganisms.Prolonged stay of tampons in the nasal cavity entails many potential complications: inflammatory changes in the middle ear and paranasal sinuses, haematympanum, acute dacryocystitis, venous stasis in the nasal mucosa, perforation of the soft palate after prolonged posterior tamponade. Absence of nasal breathing during nasal tamponade leads to a sharp decrease in partial pressure of oxygen and increased carbon dioxide content in arterial blood.Developing hypoxia can cause serious cardiovascular disorders: collapse, myocardial infarction, exacerbation of chronic thrombophlebitis of the lower extremities, pneumonia and even death as a result of obstructive sleep apnea. Cases of sepsis, meningitis, endocarditis have been described with posterior nasal tamponade. Against the background of posterior tamponade in persons with a high location of the tongue root in case of reactive oedema of the soft palate, rapidly developing hypoxia is the cause of restlessness, rise in blood pressure, renewed bleeding through the tampon and contributes to the development of DIC syndrome.

However, nasal tamponade is the most common way to stop posttraumatic, postoperative and spontaneous NK due to its availability and npocTOTbi.B.Kotechaetal (2008) conducted a questionnaire survey of 50 otorhinolaryngologists in England and Wales ^^Analysing 38 cases of treatment of NK patients, they found that in 75% of cases bleeding was stopped by anterior nasal tamponade. Surgical interventions (mainly vascular ligation) were required in less than 1% of cases, meaning that the need for them is very rare. The majority of patients with NK are treated conservatively. Similar figures are given by other authors in their works. Thus, C.Huang, C.Shu (2002) noted insufficient efficiency of tamponade only in 26.7% of patients with NK [88], D.A.Klotzetal. (2002) - y 38% [93]. Thus, in the vast majority of cases, anterior nasal tamponade is the method of choice, necessary and sufficient to stop NK.

To enhance the haemostatic effect of gauze tamponade, impregnation of tampons with various substances: aminocaproic acid, feracryl, caprofer, transamin.Aminocaproic acid blocks plasminogen activators and partially inhibits the action of plasmin, inhibits the transformation of profibrinolysin into fibrinolysin, thus inhibiting fibrinolysis. Feracryl *-1%* aqueous solution of incomplete iron salt of polyacrylic acid with iron content from 0.05 to 0.5%. The advantages of Feracryl in comparison with known haemostatic agents of local action are fast and reliable haemostatic effect, which is manifested in disorders of the coagulation system. Haemostatic effect of Feracryl is based on its ability to form water insoluble complexes with blood plasma proteins. Caprofer is a carbonyl complex of iron and aminocaproic acid. This makes it possible to prescribe it simultaneously with aminocaproic acid. When caprofera interacts with blood, a blood clot is formed, which is tightly fixed on the wound surface, preventing rebleeding. Transamine is a strong reversible monoamine oxidase (MAO) inhibitor. MAO inhibitors increase the pressor effects of sympathomimetics, which was the reason for their use as a local anaemic agent.

Unfortunately, none of the above-mentioned works has no information about the effect of the used drugs on MCT. Meanwhile, mucociliary clearance plays a leading role in the protective function of the nose and paranasal sinuses. Its disruption can subsequently lead to the occurrence of various diseases of the nose and paranasal sinuses. In this regard, in our opinion, the local application of any drug should be preceded by a study of its effect on MTT.

The absence of impaired motor function of the mesenteric epithelium is one of the advantages of the combined tampon for posterior nasal tamponade proposed by V.V. Shilenkov (2008). Shilenkov (2008) combined tampon for posterior nasal tamponade. The tampon is based on a parallelepiped wrapped with 5-8 layers of formalinised heterogeneous peritoneum. In order to enhance the haemostatic effect, the author suggested impregnating the tampon with a 20% solution of aminocaproic acid. V.V. Shilenkova noted a good haemostatic and bactericidal effect of the biological tampon, less severity of reactive inflammatory phenomena in the nasal cavity after biotamponade. Subsequently, A.V. Brofman and A.M. Gagauz (2005) used formalinised xeno-peritoneum for nasal cavity tamponade [19], and A.I. Daiches et al. (2008) used heterogeneous peritoneum preserved by freeze-drying [27]. Due to the difficulties in preparing the peritoneum for use, this method has not been widely used.

Among synthetic materials used for tamponade, foam rubber has attracted the attention of researchers. This material is elastic enough, exerts uniform pressure on tissues, and is well sterilised. It was first used for nasal cavity tamponade by I.G. Khodakov in 2000. T.Bnisis (2001) positively evaluated the gentle properties of foam rubber used for nasal tamponade, noting that it does not stick to the mucous membrane. A number of authors used the principle of Mikulich tamponade - foam swabs in glove rubber in combination with a special clip applied to the anterior parts of the nasal septum.

There are reports on the use of canoxicel and haemostatic viscose to stop NK. They are used to cut strips of the required width and wrap ordinary gauze swabs using the Mikulich principle. The resulting multilayer tampon is filled into the nasal cavity. The advantages of such a tampon are a good haemostatic effect, the presence of local antibacterial action (canoxicel contains kanamycin). In addition, canoxicel and hemostatic viscose in the presence of blood turn into an amorphous mass that can be easily removed from the nasal cavity without damaging the mucosa.

A.S. Taizhan et al. (2005) proposed to use a new sorbent tampon for anterior nasal tamponade, which consists of a moisture swelling material placed in an elastic sheath impregnated with aminocaproic acid [63]. The surface layer of the tampon is made of viscose fibre of polyolefins, which allows the contents of the nasal cavity to easily pass inside the tampon.Another way to stop NK is the use of alginate films, "Cimesol" aerosol, filling the nasal cavity with foam, merocel, hydrogels. The last two substances in contact with water increase in volume 2-3 times and are structured into gel-like state. Increase in volume while maintaining the stiffness of the material provides the action of a mechanical factor - squeezing the bleeding vessel. Statisol - aerosol also belongs to the number of haemostatic drugs that form films. After spraying in the nasal cavity, it forms an elastic film with good adhesion to the mucous membrane. The film remains on the surface of the mucous membrane for a day and provides the necessary haemostatic effect.

A number of authors express the opinion that the method of choice for stopping NK is pneumatic tamponade. A sinus catheter "Yamik" can be used as a pneumatic tampon to stop bleeding from the nasal cavity and nasopharynx. proposed by V.V.Yaroshenko and N.S.Prikhodko

(2000) pneumatic tampon allows not only to preserve nasal breathing, but also to medically affect the bleeding zone, if necessary combined with short-term hypothermia.

N.D. Timoshenko and V.I. Mahena (2001) used as a pneumatic swab an elastic tip of a medical pipette, inflated with a Politzer balloon and tied at the base with a silk thread, which is fastened around the patient's head. The pneumatic tampon has many advantages over the gauze tampon, as it is easily inserted into the nasal cavity without visual control, does not stick to the mucous membrane and is easily removed, hence does not cause repeated bleeding. At the same time, this swab has its disadvantages: more pronounced mucosal oedema and formation of widespread fibrinous plaque after removal of the swab. G.M.Klinger and R.Siegert (2007) proved by laser Dopplerography that blood flow practically stops at pressure in blood vessels of the nasal cavity mucosa exceeding 42 mmHg [92]. The pneumatic tampon proposed by Masing makes it possible to overcome a significant disadvantage of nasal tamponade - switching off nasal breathing. This tampon provides anterior and posterior tamponade, allows preserving nasal breathing, which significantly relieves the patient's condition, as it relieves from headache, dry mouth, inevitable in case of conventional tamponade. An important design feature of this tampon is the presence in the lower part of the through breathing tube with a bevel at the end, protecting the nasopharyngeal orifice of the auditory tube from damage. The breathing tube is used by many authors in various swabs.

Bleeding from the posterior nasal passages can often be stopped only by classical posterior tamponade with a gauze tampon according to Belloc, which has not been changed for several decades. In 2006, M.R. Bogomilsky and I.A. Kubylinskaya proposed tamponade of both choanas simultaneously with a single tampon, which avoids its displacement in the nasopharynx [16]. The authors use a triple catheter with one common and two separate ends. This tampon is successfully used in children with blood diseases to stop severe NK.Another modification of the posterior tampon without a third thread is proposed by the authors.

A.S. Kiselev et al. (2005) [36]. The third thread, which is withdrawn through the mouth, according to the author, traumatises the soft palate, causing the patient unpleasant sensations, especially during eating. In this case, tampon removal from the nasopharynx is performed using a curved coring rod inserted behind the soft palate.

Stopping bleeding at the site of vessel injury occurs within a certain period of time necessary for the formation of a durable thrombus. Therefore, the decision on the time of tampon stay in the nasal cavity is fundamentally important.

G.A.Gadzhimirzaev (2001) justifies the terms of tamponade taking into account pathophysiological processes occurring in the nasal mucosa [21]. At the area of contact between the tampon and damaged tissues fibrin is deposited with the subsequent formation of loose adhesions, which in 36-48 hours fix the tampon to the tissues. On the 5th-6th day fibrin lysis occurs and "oslysis" of the tampon begins. In case of tampon removal from the nasal cavity after 2 days adhesions are destroyed, which leads to recurrence of bleeding.

That is why the author proposes to remove nasal tampons on the 6th-7th day, using antibacterial therapy to prevent infection. In our opinion, unreasonable prolongation of tamponade can cause hypoxia, which is especially dangerous in patients with cerebral atherosclerosis and coronary damage. We join the opinion of SirimannaK., ToddG., MaddenG. (2007), who consider it possible to keep the tampon in the nasal cavity for no more than 48 hours [110].

The disadvantages and complications of nasal tamponade favour non-tamponade methods of treating NK.

Coagulating methods of haemostasis include chemical action on the bleeding area of the mucosa: adroxone, vagotil, trichloroacetic acid, silver nitrate; laser photocoagulation; ultrasound; argon plasma coagulation. Electrocoagulation (diathermocoagulation) and electrocaustics are the most common and available coagulating methods of stopping NK.

With the advent of endoscopic methods of investigation, the possibility of detecting the source of bleeding and direct action on it in the posterior regions of the nasal cavity has significantly increased.

Nasal endoscopy or microrinoscopy can locate and coagulate the bleeding vessel on initial presentation, saving the patient from nasal tamponade and hospitalisation.

If the bleeding site cannot be found, the entire nasal floor venous plexus is coagulated. RebeizE.E. etal., (2006) suggest coagulation of a. 8rjeporalaipaendonasal approach under endoscope control at the place of its exit through the same orifice [104].

Sharp H.R. et al. (2008) also used endoscopic endonasal coagulation of the a. sphenopalatina to stop NB [109]. This method proved to be more effective than traditional ligation of arterial vessels.Nasal bleeding can be stopped by local hypothermia.Local freezing with cryo-applicators and cryoprobes is performed with round tips inserted into the nasal cavity or by cryo-spraying.

Reactive changes after cryoapplication in the form of oedema of the nasal mucosa and the appearance of necrotic plaque persist for 1-2 weeks.

After the plaque is peeled off, the cryopreserved area is epithelialised.

The advantage of laser and cryo-intervention, according to the authors proposing to use these methods, is the absence of atrophic changes in the mucous membrane of the nasal cavity in the long term.

If conservative methods of treatment of NK do not give the desired effect, there is a need for surgical interventions, especially when the source of bleeding is located in the posterior parts of the nasal cavity.

Surgical interventions used to stop NB can be divided into 2 groups: operations in the nasal cavity, i.e., within the vascular network of the mucosa, and operations on the leading vessels.There is a report in the literature on the successful stopping of severe recurrent nasal bleeding by partial submucosal resection of the nasal septum in a child with clotting disorders due to Glanzmann's thrombasthenia gravis.

Systemic disease hereditary haemorrhagic telangiectasia (Randu-Osler Weber disease) turns out to be resistant to traditionally used surgical methods of NC treatment, including operations on the nasal septum.In the absence of nasal septum deformities, surgical detachment of the mucoperichondrium of the nasal septum completed by anterior tamponade can be used to treat recurrent NC.

One of the modern methods of ICH treatment is selective endovascular embolisation. Some authors believe that endovascular embolisation is an alternative to arterial ligations, other authors believe that endovascular embolisation is indicated only in cases when other methods of ICH arrest have proved ineffective.

Analysing the published works on the treatment of nasal bleeding, one cannot but notice that this section neglects the problem of drug treatment of NB.

There are very few special studies on conservative treatment of this pathology.

In the literature available to us, there were no recommendations for determining the indications for one or another type of replacement therapy in NK, although this is a very important issue in practical terms.

CHAPTER 2

Diangnostic methods

We examined 80 patients undergoing outpatient and inpatient treatment in the 1st and 2nd clinics of the Tashkent Medical Academy, haematology and ENT departments in the period from 2015 to 2017.

During the comprehensive examination, all patients with nasal and ONP disease combined with haematological pathology, the patients were divided into 2 groups. Group 1: 30 patients with diseases of the nose and ENP and in combination with anaemia; Group 2 - 30 patients with diseases of the nose and ENP and in combination with hemostasis pathology; and the control group consisted of 20 patients with various forms of diseases of the nose and paranasal sinuses without pathology of the blood system.

<u>**Distribution of examined patients by age and sex**</u>

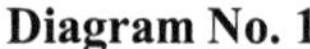

Diagram No. 1

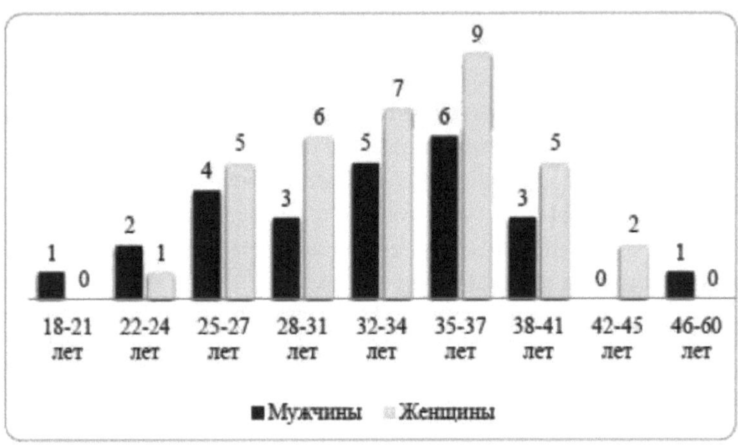

Anaemias were diagnosed based on changes in haemoglobin level, erythrocyte count, and colour index in peripheral blood of patients. The diagnosis was established on the basis of WHO recommendations (ICD10): nutrition-related anaemias (NDA), haemolytic (AIHA) and aplastic anaemias. Severe (haemoglobin level 75 g/l and below), moderate (80-100 g/l) and mild (100-110 g/l) anaemias were distinguished by severity. Of the 22 patients with severe anaemia, 12 (40%) were diagnosed with LDD, 2 (6.7%) with AIGA, 4 (13.3%) with hypo- and aplastic anaemia, and 2 (6.7%) with mixed forms of anaemia (Diagram 2).

Distribution of patients by nosological forms of anaemia.

<u>**Chart #2.**</u>

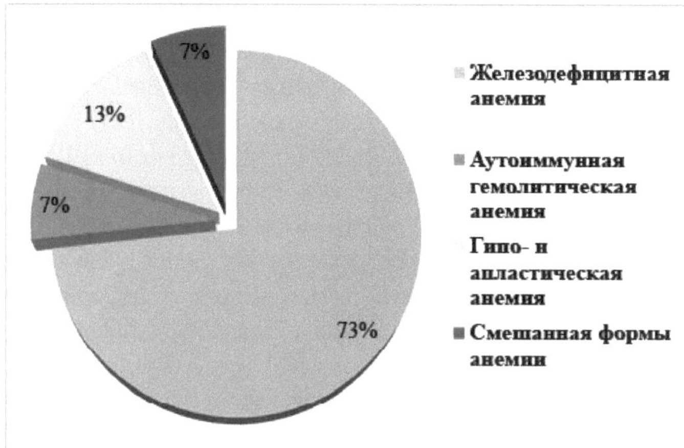

- **Iron deficiency anaemia**
- **Autoimmune haemolytic anaemia**
- **Hypo- and aplastic anaemia**
- **Mixed forms of anaemia**

The diagnosis of iron deficiency in 12 patients was established on the basis of haematological studies and ferrokinctics (determination of serum iron, transferrin, ferritin) (Table 1).

Table No. 1

Haematological parameters of patients with GDA

Indicators	WDD, n=22
Haemoglobin, g/l	68,40±1,40[a]
Erythrocytes, x10 /L[12]	2,41±0,05[a]
Colour indicator	0,64±0,01[a]
Whey iron,	6,57±0,12[a]
Ferritin, ng/ml	8,52±0,20[a]
Transferrin, g/l	4,06±0,09[a]

Note: a - differences between the indices of patients of group 1 and 3 are reliable ($P<0.05$).

The studies showed a decrease in haemoglobin level, erythrocyte content and colour index, as well as serum iron, transferrin and ferritin in the serum of the examined, which corresponds to a severe degree of WDD. This group was mainly dominated by females and of reproductive age. The clinical picture of the disease consisted of non-specific manifestations of the general anaemic syndrome (weakness, lethargy, pallor of the skin, tachycardia, dyspnoea, etc.) and manifestations of tissue iron deficiency (sideropenic syndrome). Treatment of iron deficiency was carried out against the background disease with appropriate drug correction of iron deficiency: tardiferon, sorbifer, acti- ferrin, totema, viferon, etc., taking into account sensitivity to the drug.

AIGA with acute onset ***was diagnosed in 2 patients***. The patients had darkening of urine, ictericity of sclerae and skin, fever, abdominal pain, moderate hepatosplenomegaly. Peripheral blood analysis showed a decrease in haemoglobin level (up to 41-87 g/l), erythrocyte count (up to 2.1-3.4x10^{12} /l), against the background of preservation of colour index within normal limits. Cytological analysis showed polychromasia, poikilocytosis of erythrocytes, presence of nucleus-containing erythrocytes and spherocytes. Some patients developed reticulocytosis indicators. In the bone marrow there was erythroid hyperplasia, megaloblastic type of hematopoiesis. Bilirubin content increased in serum, mainly due to indirect bilirubin. The diagnosis of AIHA was established on the basis of clinical and laboratory signs of haemolysis and the results of antiglobulin test - Coomes' test. AIHA was treated with prednisolone at a dose of 2-10 mg/kg body weight per day. In severe cases, it was combined with intravenous administration of immunoglobulin at a dose of 1 mg/kg per day.

Anaemia among the above is one of the most severe diseases of the blood system, characterised by reduction of erythroid, myeloid and megakaryocytic hematopoietic sprouts of bone marrow and pancytopenia of peripheral blood, due to defective bone marrow stem cells. The pathomorphological basis of the defect is a sharp reduction of active hematopoietic bone marrow and its replacement by fatty tissue. Out of the total number of patients with severe anaemia we examined, anaemia was diagnosed in 7 patients according to the Camita criteria (2000).

Clinical studies were carried out in 60 patients with acquired anaemia treated in the 1-2nd clinic of the Tashkent Medical Academy, haematological and ENT departments. The age of the patients was from 18 to 60 years old, and the duration of the disease was 3-26 months. The diagnosis of anaemia was established by the presence of three-growth cytopenia, anaemia, granulo- and thrombocytopenia, relative leukocytosis in peripheral blood tests and bone marrow aplasia with predominance of fatty bone marrow over active marrow in the iliac bone tri-panobioptate and myelogram. The severity of the disease was assessed by the number of granulocytes and platelets in peripheral blood (Table 2).

Table No. 2.

Peripheral blood parameters of patients with bone marrow aplasia, M±t

Indicators	Aplastic anaemia	
	non-severe, n=1	severe, n=3
Haemoglobin, g/l	50,33±1,52[a]	38,63±2,47[a]
Erythrocytes, x10 /L^{12}	2,12±0,15[a]	1,02±0,05[a]
Colour indicator	0,95±0,02	0,95±0,01
Platelets, x10 /L^{9}	42,33±4,17[a]	3,54±0,16[a]
Leukocytes, x10 /L^{9}	1,42±0,03[a]	1,01±0,02[a]
n/a neutrophils, %	1,08±0,18[a]	0,64±0,14[a]

c/e neutrophils, %	35,67±4,18[a]	20,09±1,65[a]
Eosinophils, %	1Д6±0,43[a]	1,09±0,20[a]
Lymphocytes, %	60,17±2,57[a]	69,00±1,47[a]
Monocytes, %	3,83±0,15[a]	2,91±0,16[a]
COE, mm/hour	28,67±3,88[a]	35,18±2,12[a]

Note: a - differences between the index of patients and practically healthy individuals are reliable (P<0.05).

In case of granulocytopenia less than 0.5x10^9 /L and thrombocytopenia less than 20.0x10^9 /L in combination with bone marrow aplasia according to biopsy specimens; at that bone marrow cellularity not more than 30% anaemia was diagnosed. In case of granulocytopenia more than 0.5x10^9 /L and thrombocytopenia more than 20.0x10^9 /L in combination with aplasia of bone marrow according to biopsy data, non-serious anaemia was diagnosed.

The study of peripheral blood parameters of patients with non-serious anaemia showed a reliable decrease in the content of haemoglobin, erythrocytes and platelets by 58.3; 58.3 and 91%, in sanemia patients. The content of leucocytes, paloconuclear and segmented neutrophils also significantly decreased by 69.7; 50 and 46.2% in non-serious, 78.2; 70 and 61.6%, in patients with anaemia.

Myelogram results showed a decrease in myclocytes and metamyelocytes by 53.5 and 47.4%, in paloconuclear, segmented neutrophils, eosinophils, basophils and monocytes by 57.1; 59.1; 45; 80 and 12% in nonsevere; 90 and 82%, 78.7; 80.5; 52.5; 80 and 30% in severe anaemia (Table 2.4). The content of lymphocytes and plasma cells increased sharply, exceeding the normative values by 6 and 5 times in non-severe and 7.8 and 15.3 times in severe anaemia. The content of erythroid cells was significantly low, especially in patients with anaemia. The content of megakaryocytes in patients with nonsevere anaemia decreased by 68%, and they were absent in patients with anaemia.

The disease was mainly characteristic of female individuals and was detected in all age groups. Clinical manifestations of anaemia were due to anaemic and haemorrhagic syndromes, accompanied by fever, necrotic sore throat, pronounced nasal, gingival and uterine bleeding, appearance of multiple haemorrhages on the skin and mucous membranes. (Tab.№3)

Table #3.

Myelogram parameters of patients with bone marrow aplasia, M±sh

Indicators	Aplastic anaemia	
	not heavy, =_j	severe, n=3
Myelocytes,%	4,50±0,20[a]	0,91±0,20[a]
Metamyelocytes, %	6,17±0,28[a]	2,09±0,18[a]
n/a neutrophils, %	8,17±0,28[a]	4,09±0,43[a]

c/e neutrophils, %	8,50±0,51[a]	4,09±0,39[a]
Eosinophils, %	1,83±0,15[a]	1,46±0,15[a]
Basophils, %	0,17±0,15[a]	0,09±0,09[a]
Erythroblasts, %	0,17±0,15[a]	0,09±0,09[a]
Pronormocytes, %	0,50±0,20[a]	0,0±0,0[a]
Normocytes basoph.,%	1,33±0,19[a]	0,73±0,23[a]
Polychromatophilic normocytes, %	6,00±0,24[a]	3,64±0,19[a]
Normocytes oxif.,%	1,67±0,19[a]	0,91±0,15[a]
Monocytes,%	2,17±0,15[a]	2,09±0,27[a]
Lymphocytes, %	56,83±2,40[a]	73,09±2,77[a]
Plasma cells, %	2,17±0,15[a]	3,09±0,24[a]
Megakaryocytes, /µl	3,22±0,35	Absent

Note: a - differences between the index of patients and practically healthy individuals are reliable (P<0.05).

All patients received cyclosporine A at a dose of 10 mg/kg, the duration of the course averaged 21 weeks, corticosteroids at a dose of 40 mg per day orally. 85% of patients with haemorrhagic syndrome of various severity prevailed among the examined patients, who received intensive replacement therapy with donor erythrocytes, platelets and fresh frozen plasma - 3-5 transfusions per week. In 43 (59%) anaemic patients there were infectious complications, which were treated with antibacterial, antifungal and antiviral therapy.

Idiopathic thrombocytopenic purpura was diagnosed in 2 (10%). The diagnosis of ITP was made on the basis of the following criteria: thrombocytopenia (platelets $<150X10^9$ /L) in the absence of quantitative abnormalities on the part of other blood form elements; normal or increased number of megakaryocytes in the bone marrow; absence of clinical and laboratory signs of similar disease in blood relatives; absence of clinical manifestations of other diseases or syndromes capable of causing thrombocytopenia; high level of circulating immune complexes in serum; positive effect of corticosteroid therapy. In all examined patients there were indications on haemorrhagic syndrome, nasal and gingival bleedings were manifested at the number of platelets in peripheral blood $30,0x10^9$ /l, prolongation of bleeding duration more than in 2 times (Table №4). Sufficient cellularity and normoblastic type of hematopoiesis were characteristic in bone marrow punctate.

Patients with acute and chronic ITP received glucocorticoid therapy in the form of tablets, injections and in combination, immunoglobulins for intravenous administration and cytostatic immunosuppressants, fibrinolysin inhibitors, vascular wall protectors and biological membrane stabilisers. In case of nasal haemorrhages, tampons with 5% e capric acid or dicyon were used, before that adrenaline solution in dilution 1:100000 or 1% ephedrine was injected into the nose. It was taken into account that posterior tamponade was contraindicated and anterior tamponade should be loose.

Table No. 4

Coagulological parameters of patients with thrombocytopathies, M±t

Test	ITP, n=2
Platelet count,	77,32±7,24[a]
Duration of bleeding,	208,73±6,39
Blood clotting time,	320,76±21,36
aPTT, sec	54,64±2,79
PTI, %	89,23±2,58
Fibrinogen, g/l	2,40±0,08
Thrombin time, sec	17,90±0,91

Note: reliable (P<0.05).

Various forms of thrombocytopathy were detected in 2 (10%). They were mainly characteristic of adults. Isolated and combined haemorrhages were detected with the same frequency and occurred spontaneously at any time of the day.The bleeding was mainly microcirculatory and manifested by nose and gum bleeds, anaemia of varying severity. They were characterised by a moderate decrease in platelet content, adhesion and retraction.

Haemorrhagic vasculitis was detected in 10 *(50%) of the examined patients.* The diagnosis of immune microthrombovasculitis (IMTV) was verified on the basis of analysis, clinical examination data, and laboratory results. The severity of the disease was assessed according to the criteria proposed by A.A. Ilyin. Hemostasis system indicators were characterised by preservation of normal values of platelets, clotting time, PTI and thrombin time against the background of increased fibrinogen.

Peripheral blood parameters of patients with, M±t

The content of haemoglobin, erythrocytes and platelets decreased as the disease progressed, indicating the development of severe anaemia and thrombocytopenia with the risk of hypocoagulation, especially in the blast crisis stage. The number of platelets significantly increased in 17.54; 27.51 and 28.54 times, accordingly to the stages. On this background the erythrocyte sedimentation rate increased. The main complaints of the patients were rapid fatigability, headache and dizziness, decreased appetite, nasal and gingival bleeding, heaviness in the right and left subcostals, fever and pain in the joints, temperature, the severity of which depended on the stage of the disease and duration of course. Associated pathologies were bronchopneumonia, diseases of GI, hepatobiliary and urinary systems, chronic pathologies of ENT organs, anaemia.

2.2 Methods of investigation of the examined patients.

All patients were asked in detail about their complaints and history of the disease, and the general condition of the patients was examined. When collecting anamnesis, the dates of the disease onset were clarified, the dates of recurrences, their connection with infectious diseases, respiratory system diseases, as well as the presence of an aggravated allergological anamnesis were taken into account.

Among the methods of endoscopic examination of ENT organs, the main attention was paid to anterior, middle (performed as necessary) and posterior rhinoscopy, during which all nasal cavity formations were carefully examined, as well as oropharyngoscopy, otoscopy, indirect laryngoscopy, endoscopic examination of the nasal cavity and pharynx. X-ray radiography was of great importance in the diagnosis of acute purulent sinusitis.

Radiological examination was performed in all examined patients; for this purpose, images were taken in the nasolabial, nasolabial and lateral projections. In adult patients contrast radiography was used to clarify the diagnosis. Iodlipol solution was used as a contrast agent. To clarify the prevalence of the inflammatory process some patients underwent computed tomography of the head. Particular attention was paid to the changes on the side of the eye cavity and, if necessary, ophthalmologist, neurologist, and therapist were consulted. All patients underwent general clinical analyses of blood and urine.

Rhinomanometry. In our work we used a computer rhinomanometer PC-2 (firm "Atmos" (Germany), working in the programme "Ky1po". The essence of the method consists in quantitative measurement of pressure gradient and air flow, which are created in conditions of physiological nasal breathing due to active movements of respiratory muscles. Nasal resistance indices are calculated for each half of the nasal cavity on the basis of these measurements and expressed as a fraction, in the numerator of which is a standardised pressure gradient indicator, and in the denominator is the airflow indicator. The results of rhinomanometry are given by the device in the form of a graph, and the shape of the obtained curve reflects the degree of nasal breathing disturbance.

Measurements were performed in the morning hours. The patient is in a sitting position. An adapter made of thermoplastic material is attached to the end of the pressure measuring catheter. Then the adapter together with the catheter is inserted into one of the nasal halves. The mask covers the nose and mouth, and it is suggested to perform at least four calm breathing movements. At the same time, the device registers the parameters of pressure in the half of the nose in which the catheter is inserted, as well as the air flow of the opposite half of the nose. Indicators are analysed by computer, and displayed on the monitor screen in the form of curves reflecting the inspiratory and expiratory phases. In parallel, the monitor displays quantitative indices of total volume flow (TVF) measured in cm^2 sec, total resistance (TR) to air flow at 150 Pa pressure for the left and right half of the nose in Pa/cm^2 sec. For clinical analysis, it is more appropriate to study the

summed values (SOP) and resistance (SS) for both nasal halves. The results obtained were entered into a database.
During endoscopic examinations we used rigid endoscopes of KarlStorz (Germany) with a diameter of 4.0 mm with end and side optics of 0 and 70°. The results of endoscopic examination were recorded on SonyDigitalCamera - F 828. Endoscopic examination of the nasal cavity was performed by us according to the MesserklingerW. method in the sitting position of the patient, before and after anaemisation of the nasal mucosa. All parts of the nasal cavity were examined sequentially, starting from the vestibule and nasal valve. Special attention was paid to anomalies of the middle nasal passage and nasopharynx. The middle nasal shell was examined. The examination was performed starting from its posterior end, with the endoscope moving backwards. It was possible to observe a paradoxical curvature of the middle nasal shell, which could lead to impaired ventilation of the paranasal sinuses.
The ostiomeatal complex, located in the anterior part of the middle nasal passage, is clinically important. This is the name given to the anterior ethmoidal complex in 2000 by Naumann, who defined its importance in the development of diseases of the frontal and maxillary sinus. Its components are: the anterior end of the middle shell, the hook-shaped process, the nasal tubercle cells, the semilunar cleft, the frontal pocket, the lattice bulla and the lateral sinus. Since the ostiomeatal complex contains all the natural openings of the maxillary, frontal and anterior cells of the lattice bone, it is key in the pathogenesis of acute and chronic sinusitis. The last step is to examine the upper nasal passage. Here we can examine the posterior sinus openings of the ciliary bone, the sphenoethmoidal pocket and the cuneiform sinus junction, which is located above the choanae between the nasal septum and the upper nasal shell.
With the help of a complete endoscopic examination, the causes of acute recurrent diseases of the nasal cavity and paranasal sinuses and the factors that aggravate the development of inflammation in the nasal cavity can be more accurately determined. Consequently, the choice of treatment of the disease is facilitated.
Study of mucociliary activity of the nasal mucosa
Various methods have been proposed to ***investigate the transport function of the mesenteric epithelium*** in the nasal cavity. Most of them are based on the determination of the speed of movement along the surface of the nasal mucosa of various marker particles: charcoal dust, mixture of charcoal powder with starch-agar gel, polymeric soluble film with methyl blue, black ink, blood trace.
The secretory function is based on the secretory activity of numerous mucous and serous glands, which are located in the own layer of the nasal mucosa, as well as the mesenteric cells of the epithelium. The intensity of the excretory function is determined by the amount of secretion produced by the nasal mucosa and the time

interval from the moment the film is applied to the surface of the mucosa to its complete dissolution.

The absorption ability of the nasal cavity mucosa was estimated by the degree of its staining at the location of the polymer film. The more pronounced is the suppression of motor activity of cilia, the stronger is the staining of mucous membrane with methylene blue, i.e. the better conditions for absorption are created. Absorption capacity of the mucous membrane sharply increases in atrophic processes, inhibition of cilia movement by various drugs.

In case of a sharp slowdown of mucociliary transport, strong staining of the nasal mucosa at the site of marking can be seen even during anterior rhinoscopy (Fig. 1).

Fig. No. 1

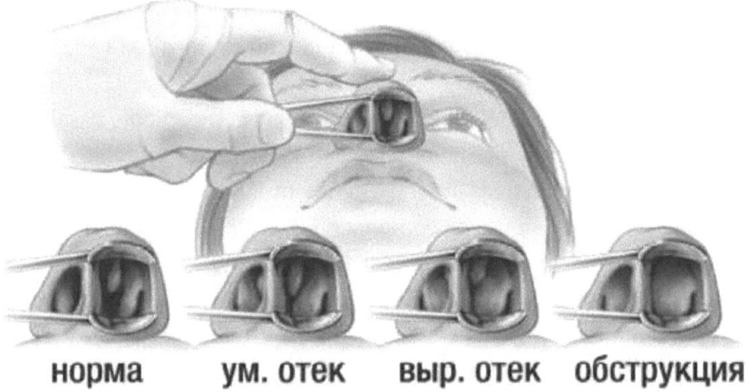

Anterior neurinoscopy.

If repeated tests confirm the immobility of the marks inserted into the nasal cavity, it can be definitively stated that this patient has a mucus transport disorder, although only electron microscopy of biopsy specimens of the nasal cavity mucosa can establish the presence of structural pathology of the cilia.Fig. №2.

Normal mucosa Virus-damaged mucosa

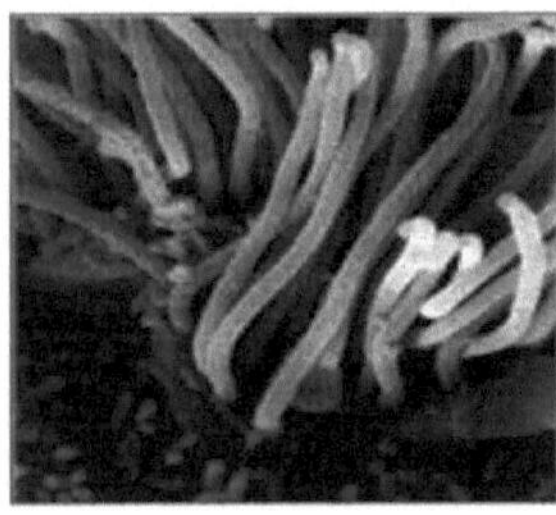

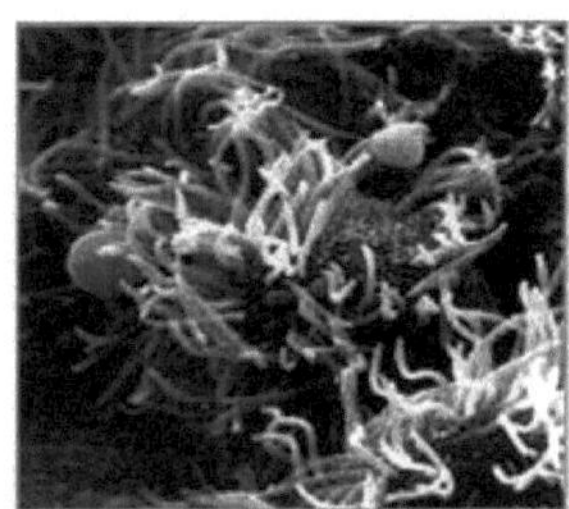

Investigation of mucociliary transport using polymer films stained with methylene blue. The film is placed on the lower nasal shell (20 minutes from the beginning of the study - the film does not dissolve, does not move, is not absorbed, which indicates a violation of MTT in a patient with deviated nasal septum and vasomotor

rhinitis).
The study of the nasal cavity calorific function was performed using a domestic electric thermometer TPEM-1 (an electric medical thermometer of the Kazan Medical Instrumental Plant) with a measuring range from 1 to 42 °C. The head of the sensor was brought to the mucous membrane of the nasal septum, at the level of the anterior end of the inferior nasal basin until light contact. The sensor head was brought to the mucous membrane of the nasal septum at the level of the anterior end of the lower nasal shell until light contact. The study was conducted in the morning hours (at 10-11 o'clock) at room temperature 18-20°C, for 20 seconds, until the complete stop of the device hand. The results of the study were recorded and entered into a computer database.
Four standard solutions were used to study the olfactory function of the nose. In ascending order of odour strength and accordingly four degrees of olfactory impairment were distinguished: 0.5 % solution of acetic acid (I degree - weak odour); pure wine alcohol (II degree - medium odour); simple valerian tincture (III degree - strong odour); ammonia alcohol (IV degree - ultra strong odour). All solution vials were of the same shape and size. Odorimetry was performed in the morning hours, before meals. The subject, was seated in front of the subject. The subject was asked to close one nostril with a finger. Dipping a piece of filter paper was brought to the open nostril, asking to smell for 2-3 seconds and identify the odorous substance, starting with acetic acid solution. Depending on the results obtained, the degree of olfactory sensitivity was established.
Bacterial examination of paranasal sinus secretionsMicrobiological studies were performed upon admission of patients to the hospital.Material for sowing was taken from paranasal sinus secretions using a bacterial loop exposed on a spirit flame. Maximum sterility was observed. Obtaining pure cultures and identification of microbes was carried out according to the rules of bacteriological technique. Purulent secretion was sown on Petri dishes with blood agar, endo medium, meat-peptone agar, Kitt-Tarotzzi medium. The growth character of microorganisms on nutrient media was determined, inherent to each culture by: shape, size, released pigment, etc. After identifying the microorganism post, a bacterial loop was contacted with the culture, which was then applied in a thin layer on the slide and spread evenly on the surface. The smears were then stained and fixed. The dried smear was viewed under immersion microscope system. The isolated strains were identified on the basis of morphological, ticcorial, culture, and biochemical properties.
Allergological study. All patients observed by us, regardless of anamnesis and complaints, were examined by an allergologist to exclude patients with allergic rhinitis from the study. Patients underwent allergological tests with bacterial and non-bacterial allergens.

CHAPTER 3

FREQUENCY AND STRUCTURE OF NASAL AND PARANASAL SINUS DISEASES IN HAEMATOLOGICAL PATIENTS

Clinical characteristics of patients

We examined 60 patients undergoing outpatient and inpatient treatment in 1-2 oy clinics of Tashkent Medical Academy haematology and ENT department for the period from2015 to2017. In the course of complex examination of 60 patients with the disease of the nose, ONP and in combination with haematological, based on the pathological process of the nasal cavity and the direction of therapeutic tactics, the patients were divided into 2 groups.

In the course of complex examination of 60 patients with nasal, ONP and in combination with haematological diseases, based on the pathological process of the nasal cavity and the direction of therapeutic tactics, the patients were divided into 2 groups.

1-group: nasal disease, ONP and in combination with haematological patients (30 patients), including 20 patients with severe anaemia, 5 patients with haemostasis pathology, 5 patients with thrombocytopenia.

2-group: nasal and ONP diseases of patients (30 patients), including 15 patients with chronic pansinusitis, 10 patients with maxillomoroethmoiditis, 5 patients with hemisinusitis. Distribution of examined patients by age and sex.

Chart #1.

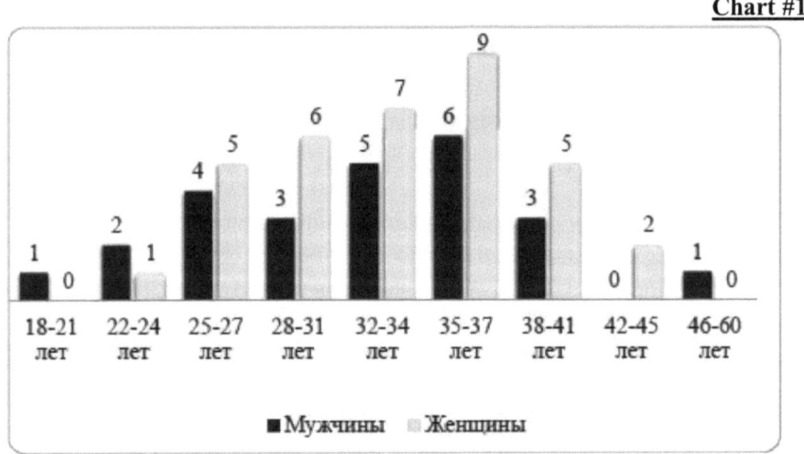

Anaemia was diagnosed on the basis of changes in haemoglobin level, erythrocyte count, and colour index in peripheral blood of patients. The diagnosis was made on the basis of WHO recommendations (ICD10):

nutrition-related anaemia (NDA), haemolytic anaemia (HCA) and aplastic anaemia. Severe (haemoglobin level 75 g/l and below, moderate (80-100 g/l) and mild (100-110 g/l) anaemias were distinguished by severity. Out of 22 patients with severe anaemia, 12 (60%) were diagnosed with LDD, 2 (6.7%) with AIGA, 4 (13.3%) with hypo and aplastic anaemia, and 2 (6.7%) with mixed forms of anaemia

(Diagram 2).

Chart #2.

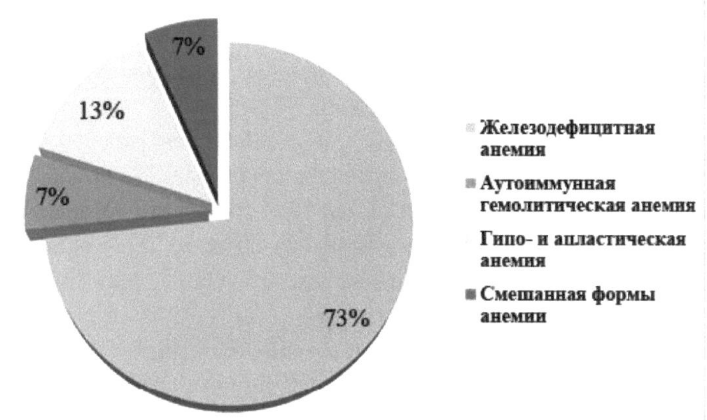

- **Iron deficiency anaemia**
- **Autoimmune haemolytic anaemia**

Hypo- and aplastic anaemia

- **Mixed forms of anaemia**

As can be seen from the above data, to a greater extent MNIONP were detected in patients with coagulopathies.

Out of 30 patients with various forms of anaemia, pathology of the ENT organs was detected. Thus, 8 patients had chronic atrophic rhinitis, 5 had simple form of chronic rhinitis, 2 had hypertrophic form, 2 had neurovegetative rhinitis and 1 had allergic rhinitis, nasal septum deviation was detected in 5 patients, and nasal bleeding of different intensity was noted in 7 patients with ENT pathology.

Diseases of the ONP were detected in 30 patients. Of these, 15 patients were diagnosed with chronic pansinusitis, 5 with chronic haimoroethmoiditis, and 5 with chronic hemisinusitis. The frequency of occurrence of various pathologies of ENT organs also depended on the age of the patient. Thus, chronic purulent middle otitis media, various forms of chronic rhinitis and sinusitis were the most frequent in 16.7% of patients, and nasal haemorrhages in 23.3%. Chronic gairomoroethmoiditis was detected in 33.3% of those examined with ENT pathology, and in all patients the process was bilateral. Chronic tonsillitis of toxic-allergic form of 1 and 11 degrees was detected in 20% of patients. Nasal bleeding, in the absolute majority of cases, was detected in hypoplastic and aplastic anaemia, while chronic inflammatory diseases of ENT organs were mainly characteristic of severe WDA.

Chronic atrophic rhinitis was mainly detected in adult patients with anaemia (26.7%). In adult patients, in contrast to children, the frequency of nasal bleeding was significantly lower and amounted to 26.7%. As in children, bleeding was mainly characteristic of aplastic anaemia, purulent-inflammatory diseases for severe GDA and mixed anaemia.According to the literature, the development of different intensity of nasal bleeding is predominantly determined by quantitative and qualitative inferiority of thrombocytopoiesis. As in children, nosebleeds were mainly characteristic of aplastic anaemia, purulent inflammatory diseases of ENT organs - for severe GAD and mixed anaemia.

Thus, based on the data obtained, we can conclude that patients with different forms of anaemia have different lesions of the ENT organs. Their nosological form and clinical manifestations depend on the type of anaemia: in aplastic anaemia, nasal bleeding of varying intensity was mainly observed, more often in children, while in severe forms of GAD and mixed anaemia - chronic purulent inflammatory diseases.

Treatment of inflammatory diseases of the maxillary sinuses.

The results of studies of the analysis of various forms of anaemia showed a variety of clinical and haematological picture and severity of syndromes. Thus, purulent-inflammatory diseases in the form of chronic purulent otitis media and pharyngitis were revealed.

More than half (6.7%) of patients with idiopathic thrombocytopenia had bleeding of varying intensity, with a higher incidence in the paediatric population. Chronic tonsillitis was detected in 23.3% of cases, which were more frequent in adults.

In patients with thrombocytopathies, bleeding of varying intensity in adults was reported in 80% of cases.

Analysis of the frequency of ENT pathologies in patients with vasculitis showed 100% occurrence of chronic tonsillitis, mainly of toxic-allergic form, as well as in adult patients. They were combined with rhinosinusitis, otitis media, rhinitis of various degrees of severity.

It is known that the development of bleeding is predominantly determined by quantitative and qualitative inferiority of thrombocytopoiesis. The severity of haemorrhagic complications coincided with the depth of thrombocytopenia. In 80% of patients with thrombocytopathies nasal bleedings of different intensity were noted, which were combined with chronic purulent-inflammatory diseases of ENT organs, chronic tonsillitis was revealed in all patients with vasculitis. Of them, in 16.7% a simple form, in 6.7% -1 degree of toxic-allergic and 6.7% - II degree of toxic-allergic form of the disease was established. 96.7% of cases were combined with sinusitis, otitis media, simple and atrophic rhinitis. Among the examined patients from all forms of chronic sinusitis there were purulent, purulent-atrophic, allergic and purulent-polyposis variants of the clinical course of the disease.

Analysis of the frequency of ENT diseases in patients with coagulopathies dictates the need for more in-depth studies of the mechanisms of their development and improvement of gentle methods of treatment.Thus, based on the obtained data, we can say that in patients with coagulopathies the frequency of ENT pathology is 76.7%, the nosological form and their manifestations depend on the form and severity of the underlying pathology.In patients with coagulopathies, the most frequent ENT diseases were nasal bleeding and chronic rhinitis.

Thus, nasal diseases in the form of various forms of acute and chronic rhinitis were detected in 5 (16.7%) and 25 (83.3%), respectively. Chronic atrophic rhinitis was diagnosed in 26.7% of patients, simple form of chronic rhinitis was detected in 16.7%, hypertrophic form - in 6.7%, neurovegetative rhinitis was noted in 6.7%, allergic form of chronic rhinitis - in 3.3% of patients. Nasal septum deviation was detected in 16.7% of patients with haemostasis pathology. Nasal haemorrhages of varying severity were noted in 23.3% of the examined patients.

Diseases of paranasal sinuses in the form of various forms of acute and chronic pathologies were detected in 5 (16.7%) and 25 (83.3%) patients. Thus, chronic pansinusitis was detected in 50% of patients, chronic gaimoroethmoiditis - in 33.3%; chronic haemesinusitis was diagnosed in 16.7% of patients.

Thus, based on the data obtained, we can conclude that diseases of the nose and paranasal sinuses were detected in 86.7% of patients with blood pathology. Two or more diseases of the nose and paranasal sinuses were diagnosed in all patients. In patients with severe anaemia diseases of nose and paranasal sinuses were detected in 86.7%, haemostasis pathology - 80% and thrombocytopenia - 6.7%. Of all diseases, nasal bleeding, atrophic rhinitis, chronic eth-moiditis, and chronic maxillary sinusitis were significantly more frequently detected.

Purulent deposits on the surface of the mucous membrane, haemorrhages, haemorrhages, intense round cell infiltration are typical for acute purulent inflammatory processes. Sometimes there were signs of peri-ostitis, rupture of the bony wall of the sinus and bleeding. Periodic or constant nasal breathing difficulty, mucous (during recurrent rhinosinusitis - mucopurulent) nasal discharge, headache, a feeling of heaviness in the forehead or cheek area, impaired sense of smell against the background of increasing rapid fatigue, drowsiness, general weakness and intoxication. It was these complaints that made them seek help from an otorhinolaryngologist.The frequency of development of various forms of sinusitis depended on the underlying pathology. Thus, anaemia was mainly characterised by purulent-atrophic chronic sinusitis (16.7%), haemostasis pathology showed all forms of sinusitis to an equal extent, amounting to 3.3%, and haemoblastosis was mainly characterised by acute and chronic purulent sinusitis (10%).

Table No. 5

Frequency of occurrence of different forms of sinusitis in haematological patients

Blood pathology	A form of sinusitis		
		Chronic	
	Acute purulent	Festering	Festering
~~Anaemia.~~	2	7	6

Pathology of haemo-	2	4	1
Trombottitope-	1	6	1

A careful history revealed a gradual onset, often after acute respiratory viral infections or after intensive polychemotherapy, with the number of recurrences increasing each year. Early complaints in this group of patients were nasal congestion, nasopharyngeal discomfort, mucous discharge from the nose and/or flowing down the posterior pharyngeal wall, and impaired sense of smell.

To objectify clinical manifestations of acute and chronic sinusitis, we used the following examination protocol (Table 6).

<u>Clinical examination protocol</u>

Table No. 6

Conversion rates:	Inspection data	
Headache: none -1, yes - 2.	General condition: satisfactory - 1, moderate - 2, severe - 3	
Diffuse -1, forehead - 2, nose - 3, occiput - 4, eyes - 5	External changes of ENT organs: none -1, deformity of the external nose - 2, adenoid face - 3	
Nasal breathing: free - 1, difficult - 2, absent - 3	Pain on palpation: frontal sinuses - 1, maxillary sinuses - 2	right to left
Nasal discharge: none -1, mucous - *2,* purulent -3	Nasal breathing: free -1, difficult - 2, absent - 3	right to left
Cough: 1 at night, 2 during the day, 3 during the day.	Nasal mucosa: unchanged -1, oedema *-2,* hyperaemia - 3	right to left
Snoring: none - 1, yes - 2.	Nasal secretion: none -1, mucus - 2, pus - 3, polyp - 4	right to left
Hearing loss: none - 1, yes - 2	Localisation of secretion in the nasal cavity: common nasal passage -1, posterior sections - 2, middle nasal passage - 3	right to left
Other complaints (specify)	Deformity of the nasal septum: none -1, ridge - 2, spike - 3, curvature - 4	Right left
Temperature (numbers): Weakness: none -1, yes - 2	Palatine tonsils: I degree -1, I degree - 2, III degree - 3	
Sick: (specify duration)	Posterior pharyngeal wall: unchanged -1, granulomatous pharyngitis - 2, lateral pharyngitis - 3, mucus - 4	right to left
Previous treatment: not treated - 1, treated as an outpatient - 2, treated as an inpatient - 3	Regional lymph nodes: not enlarged -1, painless enlarged - 2, painful enlarged - 3	right to left
What was the prior treatment:	Ears: unchanged - 1, acute purulent otitis media - 2, chronic otitis media - 3, exudative otitis media - *4*	right to left
Past illnesses:		

The common complaint of nasal breathing difficulty in 53 patients (88.3%) was common to patients of all groups. Complete absence of nasal breathing was observed in 18 patients, in 20 patients - intermittent, and in 9 patients after the use of vasoconstrictor drops nasal breathing improved for some time, but did not recover completely, and in 1 patient there was no improvement after sympathomimetics.

Next in terms of frequency of occurrence we can name headache - 42 people (70%) and rapid fatigue - 39 people (65.0%). Approximately the same prevalence of rapid fatigue in all groups probably indicates insufficient oxygen supply to the organism as a result of nasal breathing difficulties common to all patients or caused by the underlying disease.

The next most common symptom was nasal discharge in 39 patients (65%), followed by olfactory dysfunction in 21 patients (35%). These symptoms are mainly found in the group of patients with chronic rhinitis and in the group of patients with deviated nasal septum combined with rhinitis, as olfactory dysfunction of varying degrees is observed in patients with this pathology.

Nasal discharge in patients with chronic rhinitis was predominantly watery, while mucous, thick discharge was observed in patients with hypertrophic rhinitis. Purulent discharge in our patients was observed only at the time of recurrent rhinitis.

A feeling of heaviness in the cheek or forehead region in 6 people (10%), discomfort in the nasopharynx was noted by 21 people (35%). Complaints about irritability, poor appetite were intermittent.

A modified V.J. Lmid and D.W. Lmid score system was used to quantify symptoms. Lmid and D.W. Kennedy (2005), the results of which are presented in Tables 7. Quantitative assessment included the analysis of five main symptoms of the disease: nasal breathing difficulties, nasal discharge, headache, decreased sense of smell, and rapid fatigue using a two-point system; the total number could range from 10 to 10 points.

Table No. 7

Scheme for quantifying symptoms in patients with severe anaemia

Symptom	There are no Oballs	1 point sometimes, one-storey.	2points, post, bipost.	Total	Average score
Nasal breathing difficulties	25	20	27	72	1,03
Nasal discharge	26	2	44	72	1,25
Headache	36	8	28	72	0,89
Decreased sense of smell	48	3	21	72	0,63
Rapid fatigue	18	13	41	72	1,32

Total score	±5,11 0,84

Table No. 8

Scheme for quantification of symptoms in patients with thrombacyte-peniasis

Symptom	There are no Oballs	1 point sometimes, single-storey.	2-point, post, two-stor.	Total	Average score
Nasal breathing difficulties	25	20	27	72	1,03
Nasal discharge	26	2	44	72	1,25
Headache	36	8	28	72	0,89
Decreased sense of smell	48	3	21	72	0,63
Rapid fatigue	18	13	41	72	1,32
Total score					±5,11 0,84

Chart #3.

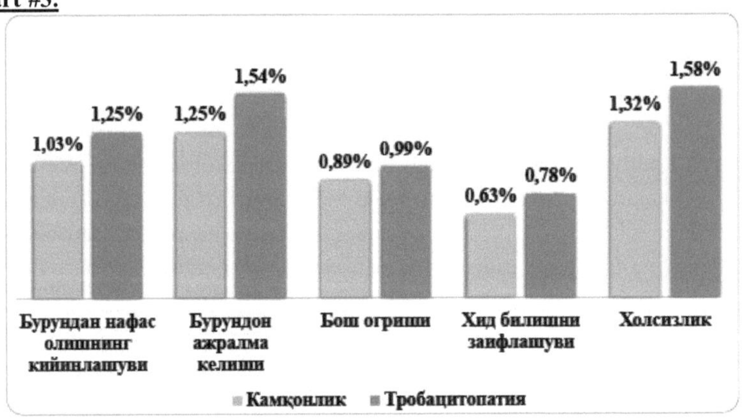

When collecting anamnesis, we asked: when the disease started, the cause of the disease, the course of the disease at the time of recurrence, and the frequency of recurrences during the year. 42(70%) patients named the known cause of the disease: colds and associated long-term use of vasoconstrictor drops, exacerbation of the underlying disease, aggressive intensive care.

One patient underwent submucosal resection of the nasal septum; about 5-6 months later, he began to experience nasal breathing difficulties and nasal discharge again. The other patient had suffered a nasal trauma. These two patients had nasal synechiae on examination and a history of frequent and prolonged colds. 7 patients underwent ultrasonic disintegration of the lower nasal shells. Two of them did not notice any improvement of nasal breathing, and the frequency of colds remained the same. In 5 patients, the condition improved and nasal breathing difficulties did not bother them for about 1.5 years, during which period the number of recurrences decreased to 2-3 episodes per year. The duration of the disease varied between groups. Overall, the group of patients with thrombacitepenia was the largest in percentage terms.

The majority of patients noted a sluggish course of the disease at the time of relapse. Only 22 (46.7%) had mild temperature reaction, the rest had no temperature reaction.The presence of concomitant allergic diseases in patients, such as bronchial asthma, urticaria, migraine, allergic conjunctivitis, allergic dermatitis, was revealed in 3.3% of cases (4 patients).In groups of patients with combined pathology, chronic bronchitis took the first place. In 23.3% of patients with a history of pneumonia, and in 10% of patients pneumonia was diagnosed more than once.Thus, anamnestic data provide a sufficiently complete assessment of the patient's general state of health.The data of endoscopic examination of the nasal cavity showed the following (Table 9).

Nasal cavity endoscopic findings in haematological patients

Table 9

sign	Number of cases
Hyperaemia and swelling of the nasal mucosa	22
Deformity of the nasal septum	8
Hypertrophy of the lower nasal bones	24
Pathological discharge	17
Synechiae	2
Pathology of the middle nasal shell	9
Hypertrophy of the lattice bulla	9
Hypertrophy of the hook-shaped process	3

Nasal septal deviation was detected in 8 patients, which was 26.7%. In 7 patients a nasal septal tubercle was detected during endoscopic examination, and in 12 patients pronounced ridges were observed. Endoscopic examination is of great importance to investigate the posterior septum.

Examination before anaemisation in 22 patients revealed hyperaemia of the nasal mucosa. In 30 patients hypertrophy of the lower nasal shells was detected, in 24 patients after anaemisation the posterior end of the lower nasal shells did not contract, and in 4 patients after anaemisation the lower nasal shells remained unchanged; Hypertrophic rhinitis is characterised by purple-red colouring of the mucous membrane of the nasal cavity. In the cavernous form of hypertrophic rhinitis the surface of the nasal shells is smooth, even, in fibrotic - areas of smooth surface alternate with areas of mucosa covered with papillae, which are most often observed either at the ends of the shells, or along their lower edge, usually on the lower nasal shell. Scanty or moderate mucous discharge without paroxysms of rhinorrhoea, usually viscous, the amount of which for a long time is constant, in some patients with hypertrophic rhinitis may be absent at all. When probing the surface of the shell after adrenalisation, in the cavernous form of hypertrophic rhinitis, its bony base is noted; in the fibose form, the overgrown dense connective tissue reduces the sensation of bone. Dense tissue of the mucous membrane is felt, the probe is not pressed into it and does not leave a groove behind it. In vasomotor rhinitis due to oedema of nasal shell tissues, the probe easily passes deep into the tissue and rests on the bone. After removal of the probe in this place leaves an indentation, which gradually smoothes out. For vasomotor rhinitis is characterised by swelling of the mucous membrane of the nasal cavity up to complete obstruction of its lumen with the simultaneous appearance of copious amounts of mucus or watery discharge, the colour of the mucous membrane is quite different - pink and blue. Sometimes we can observe a rapid change of colour from bright red to brown with the appearance of signs of vascular dystonia - Voyachek's spots. After anaemisation (lubrication of the mucous membrane with 0.1% adrenaline solution) the nasal shells shrank and took normal size.

Pathology of the middle nasal shell: pathologically curved middle nasal shell was found in 9 cases, bullous hypertrophy of the middle nasal shell - in 9 patients. 9 patients had bul- laethmoidalis, which partially blocked the junction of the maxillary sinus. In all these patients the dominant complaint was difficulty of nasal breathing mainly on the same side.Progression of chronic leukaemia was accompanied by an increase in the frequency of complaints, an increase in objective symptomatology. The picture of concomitant pathology of ENT organs had a vague clinical manifestation.

In the study of functional characteristics of the nasal cavity mucosa, the norm indicators of transport, excretory and suction functions were determined. As indicated above, this study was carried out on healthy individuals. In addition, the average values of the main indicators in patients with recurrent sinusitis depending on the nature of the lesion of intranasal structures were determined.

During the saccharin test before surgery, the saccharin time was significantly longer in all patients than in the control group, which is most likely due to the pathology of intranasal structures (standard deviation was 6.4 min). Slowdown of mucociliary transport promotes a longer contact of viruses and bacteria with the epithelium, which predisposes to the development of the inflammatory process.

The results of the study are presented in Table 10. The results of the study allowed us to conclude that the functional abilities of the mesenteric epithelium are most reduced in the group of patients with combined pathology of the nasal cavity.

Table 10.

Assessment of functional abilities of the nasal mucosa in patients with recurrent rhinosinusitis and in healthy individuals.

sign	Functions of the mucous membrane of the nasal cavity		
	Transport (min.)	Excretory (min.)	Suction
Vasomotor rhinitis	42,1+0,2*	4,6±0,2*	strong colouration
KO hypertrophy combined with vasomotor rhinitis	43,4+0,7*	5,1±0,2*	strong colouration
NP deformity combined with vasomotor rhinitis	45,4+0,4*	6,4±0,5	strong colouration
Hypertrophic rhinitis	38,2+0,3*	5,4±0,4*	moderate colouration
SR pathology combined with NP deformity and hypertrophic rhinitis	44,3+0,3*	6,9±0,5	strong colouration
Laryngeal bulla hypertrophy combined with NP deformity and hypertrophic rhinitis	47,5+0,3*	5,6±0,3*	strong colouration
Synechiae	35,4+0,1*	4,3±0,1*	moderate colouration
Norma	24,1+1,2	8,12+0,3	moderate colouration

Note: NP - nasal septum, SR - middle bulb,
KO is the hook-shaped process.

Chart #4.

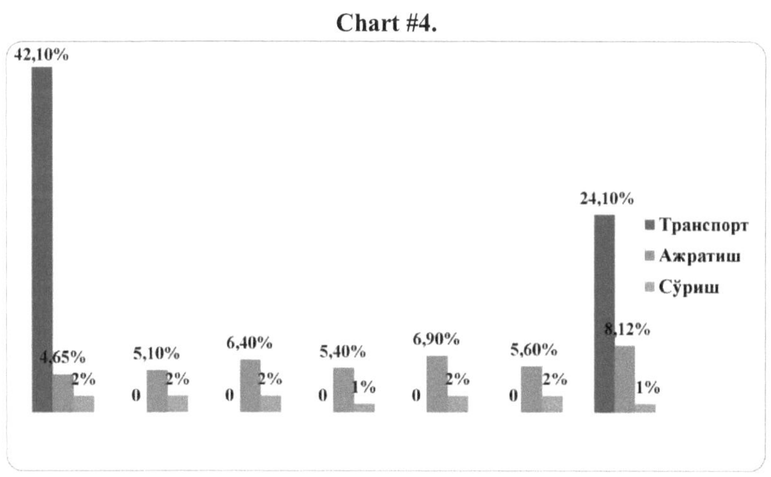

Based on these data, we can conclude that the cause of recurrent inflammatory diseases in patients with anatomical anomalies of the nasal cavity is a violation of the interaction between the mucociliary and immune defence systems. As a consequence, we observe: firstly, an increase in the severity and duration of acute infectious diseases, secondly, a significant bacterial contamination of the nasal mucosa, leading to a further increase in the frequency of recurrences. Therefore, traditional drug treatment, as a rule, is successful only in exacerbations, but does not prevent relapses.

In all patients, the species composition of microflora isolated from the nasal cavity mucosa from under the middle nasal shell during the interrelapse period and from the punctate of maxillary sinuses at the time of purulent inflammation, as well as its sensitivity to antibiotics were determined.When studying the microflora detected from the punctate of maxillary sinuses (Table 3. 3.8), the following results were obtained: the most frequently isolated flora was Hemophilusinfluenza (12.2%), Staphylococcusaureus (5.7%), Hemophilusparainfluenzae (5.7%), Staphylococcusepidermidis (4.1%), M.catarrhalis (7.3%) detected in 42 cases (34.1%). Absence of microflora was noted in 17 cases (13.8%) Monocultures were isolated in 60 patients (85.4%): Streptococcuspneumoniae (36.2%), Streptococcuspyogenes (24.8%), Staphylococcuspyogenes (24.8%), Staphylococcus cusaureus (14.3%), Hemophilusinfluenza (9.5%), Staphylococcusepidermidis (5.7%), Hemophilusparainfluenzae (4.8%), M.catarrhalis (4.8%). Microbialassociation was isolated in 9 (7.3%) patients: S.pneumoniaeH.influenzae4 patients; H.influenzaeStreptococcuspyogenes3 patients; H.parainfluenzaeStreptococcuspyogenes2 patients.The most frequently isolated pneumococcus (Streptococcuspnemnoniae) was 42 cases (34.1%).

Chart #5.

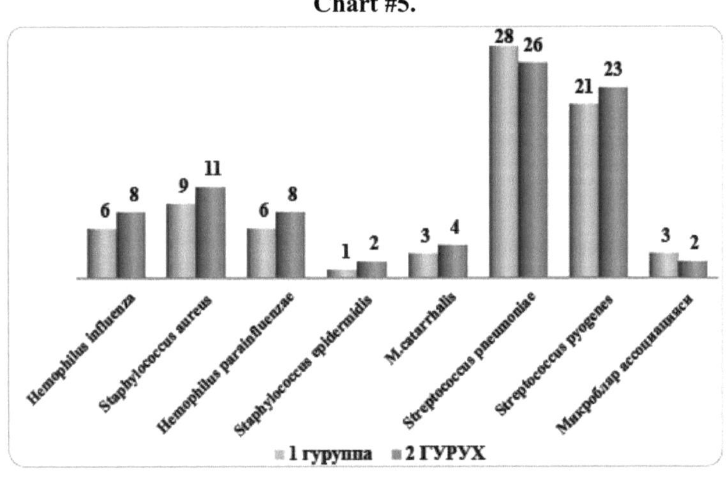

The study of the species composition of microflora isolated from the nasal mucosa of patients with recurrent rhinosinusitis revealed the predominance of gram-positive microflora (Staphylococcusepidermidis, Streptococcuspneumoniae,

Streptococcusviridians, Staphylococcusaureus). Analysing the obtained data, we came to the conclusion that the most common bacterial microflora in all patients suffering from recurrent rhinosinusitis is Staphylococcusepidermidisó00 patients (55.3%). In 40.65% of cases Staphylococcusaureus can be detected***(30 patients***).

According to the literature, Staphylococcusaureus is a pathogenic flora and has a pronounced sensitising property. When it interacts with the human body, immediate and delayed hypersensitivity reactions occur. Toxins derived from epidermal and Staphylococcus aureus depress the motor activity of the mesenteric epithelium; the greatest degree of inhibition of secretion transport is observed under the influence of Staphylococcus aureus causing haemolysis of erythrocytes. Staphylococcusaureus is often combined with Streptococcus and pneumococcus, usually as an expression of mixed infection.

In the group of healthy patients, Staphylococ- cusepideraiidis was isolated in 70% of cases, and in 5% of cases -Streptococcusviridans. That is, in healthy people opportunistic flora, in this case greening streptococcus, is rare. The absence of microflora was found in 25%. It was found that the antibiotics to which the microflora isolated from the nasal mucosa of patients was sensitive were amoxicillin clavulanic acid, cefotaxime, fluoroquinolone preparations. Amoxicillin clavulanic acid is a penicillin drug of the penicillin series with clavulanic acid, which provides protection against the hydrolysing enzyme B-lactamase. It has a broad spectrum of action with a greater focus on suppression of triple for respiratory tract microorganisms Streptococcusp neumoniae and Haemophilusinfluenzae. Particularly pathogenic flora (Pseudomonasaerugenosa, Proteusvulgaris, E.coli, Citrobacterfreundii, found highly resistant to many antibiotics, including 3rd generation cephalosporins Cefotaxime 1.0), importantly, was highly sensitive to fluoroquinolone series drugs (Levofloxacin 100.0).

Thus, the causative agent of the disease is mainly microflora isolated from the punctate of the maxillary sinus.

A significant bacterial contamination of the nasal mucosa (including the presence of Gram-negative opportunistic microflora with a wide spectrum of resistance to antibiotics) gives reason to attribute it to the risk factors for the formation of secondary local immune insufficiency and persistence of the inflammatory process in patients with anatomical anomalies of the nasal cavity.

However, the clinical picture of purulent-inflammatory diseases of ENT organs depended on the course of the underlying pathology. Thus, in patients with a severe degree of LDD, aplastic anaemia and autoimmune haemolytic anaemia, simple and atrophic forms of chronic rhinitis and pharyngitis, simple and I degree of toxic-allergic forms of chronic tonsillitis and chronic meso-tympanitis were detected in various combinations. Among the examined patients from all forms of chronic sinusitis there were purulent and purulent-atrophic variants of the clinical course of

the disease. The clinical picture of chronic sinusitis varied from the clinical form and stage of the disease. The amount of discharge was determined by the patency of the sinus outlet, as well as by the number of paranasal sinuses involved in the pathological process. The clinical picture of purulent atrophic rhinitis and sinusitis was characterised by less pronounced clinical signs of the inflammatory process. The mucous membrane of nose and nasal passages were atrophic, thin, difficult to separate purulent discharge was scanty with sharp odour and sometimes in the form of crusts, there was dryness of mucous membranes of nose and perinasal passages. In chronic purulent middle otitis media (mesotympanitis) subjective symptoms were weakly expressed. The main complaints of patients are purulent flow from the ear and lowering of ear
hearing. Odourless oesophageal and purulent discharge. Perforation of the tympanic membrane of different size and configuration, not marginal. In microbiological examination there was a predominance of isolation of several microorganisms, often anaerobes. At the same time, chronic sinusitis proceeded in the form of purulent inflammation, inert, poorly amenable to treatment, often accompanied by nasal bleeding.

Consequently, inflammatory diseases of paranasal sinuses in patients with anaemia proceed with a pronounced shift of haematological indicators of intoxication of the organism, increasing auto-intoxication, hypoxia, overstrain of adaptation mechanisms and transition of adaptation-compensatory immunological reactions to damaging ones.

Analysing the obtained data, it should be said that most anaemias have systemic lesions of all organs and systems. First of all, this is due to a sharp change in the immunological properties of the body, homeostasis disorders, suppression of the detoxification system organs, disruption of central and peripheral haemodynamics, causing the development of hypoxia. This contributes and widely used chemotherapeutic treatment, especially in aplastic and mixed anaemia. Existing in the pathology of the blood system, the above changes may cause a violation of the mucous membrane of the upper respiratory tract, slow down the processes of their repair and reduce their resistance to infection. It is known that any infection against the background of altered immunobiological reactivity of the organism, creates a "vicious circle".

Based on the studies of patients with severe forms of anaemia, it can be said that the underlying pathology imposes a certain imprint on the clinical course of diseases of the nose and paranasal sinuses:

- predominance of local symptoms over general symptoms, among the complaints - flow of discharge into the nasopharynx for a long time, fever and cough;

in anaemia rhinoscopically, sinusitis was characterised by scant objective symptomatology;

- inflammatory diseases of the paranasal sinuses proceed with pronounced intoxication of the body.

Of these, 48% had a simple form, 37% had grade 1 toxic-allergic and 15% had grade II toxic-allergic forms of the disease. 49% of cases were combined with sinusitis, otitis media, simple and atrophic rhinitis. Among the examined patients from all forms of chronic sinusitis there were purulent, purulent-atrophic variants of clinical course of the disease. The clinical picture of chronic sinusitis varied from the clinical form and stage of the disease. The amount of discharge was determined by the patency of the sinus outlet, as well as by the number of paranasal sinuses involved in the pathological process. The clinical picture of purulent otitis media was characterised by otorrhea and hearing loss. Perforation of tympanic membrane of different sizes and configurations. In the course of treatment the diseases were difficult to be treated with antibiotics.

Based on the studies of patients with haemostasis pathology, it can be said that the underlying pathology imposes a certain imprint on the clinical course of diseases of the nose and paranasal sinuses:

- frequent recurrent haemorrhage with massive blood loss;
- manipulations of the nasal cavity (puncture and probing of the sinuses, Proitz nasal lavage, etc.) are accompanied by bleeding;
- inflammatory diseases of the paranasal sinuses proceed with pronounced intoxication of the body.

However, dystrophic changes of the nasal cavity mucosa in the area of ridges and spines of the nasal septum were observed in all cases. Dystrophic changes of the nasal cavity mucosa, mainly in the anterior parts, were detected in 25 (46.3%) patients. In patients with anterior dry rhinitis the common complaints were discomfort, dryness and itching in the nose, crust formation.

In microbiological examination there was a predominance of isolation of several microorganisms, often anaerobes. At the same time, chronic sinusitis proceeded in the form of purulent inflammation, inert, poorly amenable to treatment, often accompanied by nasal bleeding. Isolated lesions of one sinus were detected in 10% of patients, poly, hemi and pansinusitis were detected in 58; 10 and 22% of patients.

When examining patients with thrombocytopenia (35.5% of cases), acute pathology of ENT organs, etiologically related to the development of the underlying disease, as well as naturally occurring in the course of treatment of the underlying disease, was detected: NK, acute rhinitis and inflammatory diseases of the ENP, furuncles of the nose and nasolabial triangle, herpes of the skin and mucous membranes of ENT organs.

In haematological patients with concomitant pathology of ENT organs (acute purulent sinusitis, otitis media, tonsillitis) there is a rapid manifestation of intoxication of the body, characteristic local changes, etc. Typical for acute purulent-inflammatory processes are purulent deposits on the surface of the mucous membrane, haemorrhages, haemorrhages, intense round cell infiltration.

The progression of chronic leukaemia was accompanied by an increase in the frequency of complaints and an increase in objective symptoms. The picture of concomitant pathology of ENT organs had a sterile clinical manifestation. Chronic tonsillitis, pharyngitis, severe abscesses of the nasal septum, etc. were detected.

Conclusion

1. In patients with nasal cavity pathology, mucociliary transport, excretory and absorptive function of the nasal mucosa is slowed down.
2. The study of the species composition of microflora isolated from the nasal mucosa of patients with recurrent rhinosinusitis revealed the predominance of Gram-positive microflora (Staphylococcus epidermidis, Streptococcus pneumoniae, Streptococcus viridians, Staphylococcus aureus).
3. A 70% positive result was obtained in patients with blood diseases when combined antibiotics were used in the effective treatment of rhinosinusitis.

Literature

1. Abdulkadyrov K.M. Haematology (reference book).- SP 5 2004 - 928 p.
2. Abdulkadyrov K.M. Bessmeltsev S.S. Aplastic anaemia - SP 6 2006 - 232 pp.
3. Aksenov V.M., Pakhomov I.L., Chifligarova T.V., Sinebogov S.V. Nasal haemorrhages and modern methods of their stopping Vesti. Otorinolar.
- 2004 - №4 - c. 33-34.
4. Alerdot L.M. Unresolved problems in the treatment of haemophilia Herald of Blood Service of Russia. 2000 -№5-C 80-84.
5. Amonov Sh.E., Vesti. TMA: -2010 -#2. pp. 78-80.
9. Arkhipova Y.V., The role of ***dysaggregation thrombocytopathies in the occurrence of haemorrhagic complications in rhinology.*** //Ross.rhinologiya-2005 - №2 -.
C.31-32.
10. Atlas. Computed tomography in diseases of the nasal cavity, paranasal sinuses and ear. Moscow, 2016 -65 pp.
11. Atlas of haematology. Shawna K. Anderson, Kayla B. Poulsen - Moscow, 2007-453 p.
12. Bargakan Z.S. Momot A.P. DHS-syndrome and thrombocytopenic purpura in oncohematological diseases. Problems of clinical medicine - 2005- №1-C.22-24.
13. Baryshev B.A. *Place of Tachocomb among traditional methods of local* haemostasis. Tachocomb - five-year experience of application in Russia: collection of articles - Moscow, 2001 - P. 8-12.
14. Batrak T.A. Participation of fibrin monomer polymerisation disorders in the genesis of various types of bleeding : autoref. Doctor of Medical Sciences - Barnaul, 2000 - 32 p.
15. Bogomilsky M.R., Garashchenko T.P., Nasal haemorrhages in children with thrombacitepenia Vesti. Otorinolar. 2003.
16. Bogomilsky M.R., Kubylinskaya I.A. Modification of posterior tamponade for nasal bleeding in children with thrombacitepenia Vesti, otorinolar. - 2006 -№3 - c. 49.
17. Bogomilsky M.R., Chistyakova V.R., 2005 Treatment of recurrent inflammatory diseases of the nasal cavity and paranasal sinuses. //Autoref. dissertation, Candidate of Medical Sciences.
Moscow, 2008
18. Boyko N.V. To pathogenesis of nasal bleeding recurrences Russian rhinology - 2000 - №3 - p. 39-44. 39-43.
19. Brofman A.V., Gagauz A.M. Application of formalinised xenobrews for stopping nasal bleeding allo and xenogenic material in transplantation - Chisinau, 2005 - pIb-118.
20. Byrikhina V.V. 2007 Vinogradova M.A., Klyasova G.A., Trushina E.E. et al. Infectious complications in the debut of aplastic anaemia. Haematol i transfusiol -

T. 52. №4-C. 16-21.

21. Gadzhimirzaev G.A. Methods of drainage and tamponisation in otorhinolaryngological practice Vesti, otorhinolary - 2001 - №6. p. p. 44-44. 44-47.

22. Karpov V.A., Nasal haemorrhage and endonasal surgical methods of its stopping. Kiev 2004 - 95 p.

23. Kiselev A.S. Treatment of acute and recurrent exudative sinusitis after ineffective systemic antibiotic therapy: Methodical manual for doctors. Yaroslavl, 2005 - 43 pp.

24. Kovaleva L.M., Foschan A.V., Sinusitis: a modern view of the problem // Sop siliummedicum, 2016,- Vol. 5,- No. 4,- P.212-218.

25. Kozlov V.S. Haemodynamics of the mucous membrane of the nasal cavity, nasal breathing and mucociliary transport in norm and pathology. Otorinolar - 2003 - № 6 - p.38-40.

26. Kozlov V.S., Markov G.I., Treatment and diagnostic tactics for nasal bleeding in patients with acute leukaemia // Herald of Otorhinolaryngology - 2010 - No.1 - P.51-54

27. Kozlov V.S. Shilenkova V.V. Ultrasonic diagnostics of perinasal sinus diseases. M- 2007- P.75-83.

28. Kuznetsov S.V., Nakatis J.A., Application of polyvinyl pyrrolidone films for tamponade of the nasal cavity //Vestnik otorhinolaryngologii 2012. No. le. 28-30.

29. Kurilin I.A. Rogozhin V.A. Sudoma A.S. Prospects for the use of computed tomography in otorhinolaryngology ZHUNGB - 2015-#4 -C. 6
11.

30. Lavrenova G.V. et al, Aplastic anaemia: immunopathogenesis, clinic, diagnostics, treatment - Novosibirsk: Nauka. - 2003 -212 c.

31. Limansky S.S., Kondrasheva O.V. Treatment of recurrent inflammatory diseases of the nasal cavity and paranasal sinuses. //Autoref. diss.k.m.n. Moscow, 2005

32. BetaL., Sprekelsen M, Simultaneous inferior and middle meatus antrostomies in the treatment of the severely diseased maxillary sinus. //Am. J. Rhinol. Allergy- 2009 - Vol. 3.

33. Borts M.R., Druce H.M., Developmental hemostasis: Relevance to hemostatic problems during childhood //Tromb. Hemostasis 2013 - Vol. 21, N4-P 341-356.

34. Bnisis THeat shock genesintegrating Cell, survival and death //J. Biosci - 2001 - Vol. 32 - P 595-610.

35. Clemans D.L et al. Ear. Nose.and throat diseases. A pocket reference. Second edition - Stuttgart - New York: Thieme, 2008.

36. Clement P.A., et al., et al. Effects of simulated bleeding in an in vitro nasal fibroblast wound healing model. // Rhinol Allergy - 2006 - Vol 24(3) -P 186-191.

37. Clement P.A., Haemophilias A and B //Lancet. 2009. - Vol. 361,N9371.-P. 180-180.

38. DavidsonTet al The usefulness of the Platelia Candida antigen in a patient with acute lymphocytic leukaemia and chronic disseminated candidiasis. //Med. Mycol - 2006 - Vol. 44(7) - P 647-650.

39. Fireman P., Pathological mechanisms and clinical features of eosinophilic chronic rhinosinusitis in the Japanese population. //Allergol Int- 2002- Vol 59(3)- P 247-256.

40. Fokkens W et al: Efficacy of ice packs in the management of epistaxis //Clin. Otolaryngol. Allied Sc. 2007 - vol. 28(6) - pp 545-7

41. Glasier C.M. et al, White P. Routine coagulation screening in the management of emergency admission for epistaxis - is it necessaiy H J. Laryngol. Otol - 2002 - vol. 114(1) - pp 38-40.

42. Gliklich R. E., Metson R et al. Reliability of EP30S symptom criteria and nasal endoscopy in the assessment of chronic rhinosinusitis - a GA (2) LEN study // Allergy- 2005- Vol.17- P. 95-99.

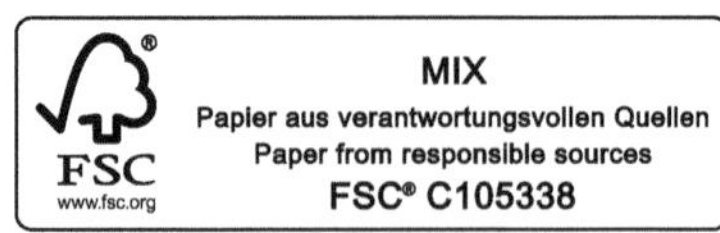

Printed by Books on Demand GmbH, Norderstedt / Germany